Gastrointestinal Physiology

Look for these other *Mosby Physiology Monograph Series* titles:

Blankenship: NEUROPHYSIOLOGY (978-0-323-01899-9)

Blaustein et al: CELLULAR PHYSIOLOGY (978-0-323-01341-3)

Cloutier: RESPIRATORY PHYSIOLOGY (978-0-323-03628-3)

Koeppen & Stanton: RENAL PHYSIOLOGY, 4TH EDITION (978-0-323-03447-0)

Levy & Pappano: CARDIOVASCULAR PHYSIOLOGY, 9TH EDITION (978-0-323-03446-3)

Porterfield & White: ENDOCRINE PHYSIOLOGY, 3RD EDITION (978-0-323-03666-5)

Gastrointestinal Physiology

SEVENTH EDITION

Edited by

LEONARD R. JOHNSON, PhD

Vice Chancellor for Research
Thomas A. Gerwin Professor of Physiology
University of Tennessee Health Sciences Center
Memphis, Tennessee

MOSBY

ELSEVIER

MOSBY
ELSEVIER

1600 John F. Kennedy Blvd.
Ste 1800
Philadelphia, PA 19103-2899

GASTROINTESTINAL PHYSIOLOGY ISBN-13: 978-0-323-03391-6
Copyright © 2007 by Mosby, Inc., an affiliate of Elsevier Inc. ISBN-10: 0-323-03391-1

Notice

Knowledge and best practice in this field are constantly changing. As new research and experience broaden our knowledge, changes in practice, treatment, and drug therapy may become necessary or appropriate. Readers are advised to check the most current information provided (i) on procedures featured or (ii) by the manufacturer of each product to be administered, to verify the recommended dose or formula, the method and duration of administration, and contraindications. It is the responsibility of the practitioner, relying on their own experience and knowledge of the patient, to make diagnoses, to determine dosages and the best treatment for each individual patient, and to take all appropriate safety precautions. To the fullest extent of the law, neither the Publisher nor the Editor assumes any liability for any injury and/or damage to persons or property arising out of or related to any use of the material contained in this book.

The Publisher

Previous editions copyrighted 1977, 1981, 1985, 1991, 1997, 2001

Library of Congress Cataloging-in-Publication Data
Gastrointestinal physiology / edited by Leonard R. Johnson.—7th ed.
   p. ; cm.
  Includes bibliographical references and index.
  ISBN-13: 978-0–323–03391–6   ISBN-10: 0–323–03391–1
    1. Gastrointestinal system—Physiology. 2. Digestion. I. Johnson, Leonard R.,
  [DNLM: 1. Digestive Physiology. WI 102 G2571 2007]
  QP145.G27 2007
  612.3—dc22   2006041999

Acquisitions Editor: William Schmitt
Developmental Editor: Kevin Kochanski
Publishing Services Manager: Linda Van Pelt
Project Manager: Francisco Morales
Design Direction: Lou Forgione

ISBN-13: 978-0–323–03391–6
ISBN-10: 0–323–03391–1

Printed in China

Last digit is the print number: 9 8 7 6 5 4 3 2

CONTRIBUTORS

LEONARD R. JOHNSON, PhD
Vice Chancellor for Research
Thomas A. Gerwin Professor of Physiology
University of Tennessee Health Sciences Center
Memphis, Tennessee

NORMAN W. WEISBRODT, PhD
Professor and Chairman
Department of Integrative Biology and Pharmacology
University of Texas Medical School
Houston, Texas

PREFACE

The first edition of *Gastrointestinal Physiology* appeared in 1977. It developed as a result of the authors' teaching experiences and the need for a book on gastrointestinal physiology written and designed for medical students and beginning graduate students. This seventh edition is written by the same authors and directed to the same audience. As with any new edition, those involved usually believe that it is significantly better than the previous one. Dr. Weisbrodt and I feel strongly that this edition is such an improvement. All chapters contain significant amounts of new material and have been brought up-to-date with current information, without introducing undue amounts of controversy to confuse students.

There are two major changes in the seventh edition. The chapter on the splanchnic circulation has been dropped. This material usually is covered in cardiovascular texts and is taught as part of cardiovascular physiology in most courses. A new chapter on the regulation of food intake has been added. Although our information on this subject is far from complete, obesity is fast becoming the number one health problem in the developed world. We therefore feel it is important that students begin to develop an understanding of this field. The entire book is still written by the original authors. I am indebted to Dr. Weisbrodt for his continuing contributions and ability to transmit his expertise in a lucid and concise manner. As always, I also am grateful that his revised chapters arrived on schedule so that our publishing deadline could be met.

We are grateful to our own students for pointing out ways to improve the book. Numerous colleagues in other medical schools and professional institutions have added their suggestions and criticisms as well. We are thankful for their interest and help, and we hope that anyone having criticisms of this edition or suggestions for improving future editions will transmit them to us.

We would like to thank H.J. Ehrlein and Michael Schemann for generously allowing us to link the videos referenced in Chapters 4 and 5, which appear on the website of the Technische Universität München (http://www.wzw.tum.de/humanbiology/data/motility/34/?alt=english). The videofluoroscopy on gastrointestinal motility of dogs, pigs, and sheep was performed during the scientific studies of H.J. Ehrlein and his colleagues over a period of 25 years. This video project was supported by an educational grant from Janssen Research Foundation.

Finally, I thank Ms. Easter Jenkins for typing my own chapters and helping with the communications and organizational work that are a necessary part of such a project.

LEONARD R. JOHNSON

CONTENTS

CHAPTER 1

REGULATION: PEPTIDES OF THE GASTROINTESTINAL TRACT 1

LEONARD R. JOHNSON

General Characteristics   1
Discovery   2
Chemistry   3
Distribution and Release   5
Actions and Interactions   6
Candidate Hormones   8
Neurocrines   9
Paracrines   10
Clinical Applications   10
Clinical Tests   11
Summary   11
Key Words and Concepts   11

CHAPTER 2

REGULATION: NERVES AND SMOOTH MUSCLE 13

NORMAN W. WEISBRODT

Anatomy of the Autonomic Nervous
    System   13

Neurohumoral Regulation of Gastrointestinal
    Function   15
Anatomy of the Smooth Muscle Cell   16
Smooth Muscle Contraction   17
Summary   20
Key Words and Concepts   21

CHAPTER 3

SWALLOWING 23

NORMAN W. WEISBRODT

Esophageal Peristalsis   23
Receptive Relaxation of the Stomach   28
Clinical Applications   28
Clinical Tests   29
Summary   29
Key Words and Concepts   30

CHAPTER 4

GASTRIC EMPTYING 31

NORMAN W. WEISBRODT

Anatomic Considerations   31
Contractions of the Orad Region of the
    Stomach   32
Contractions of the Caudad Region of the
    Stomach   32

Contractions of the Gastroduodenal
Junction   34

Contractions of the Proximal
Duodenum   34

Regulation of Gastric Emptying   35

Clinical Applications   37

Clinical Tests   38

Summary   38

Key Words and Concepts   38

CHAPTER 5

MOTILITY OF THE SMALL INTESTINE ... 41

NORMAN W. WEISBRODT

Anatomic Considerations   41

Types of Contractions   41

Patterns of Contractions   42

Clinical Applications   46

Clinical Tests   46

Summary   47

Key Words and Concepts   47

CHAPTER 6

MOTILITY OF THE LARGE INTESTINE ... 49

NORMAN W. WEISBRODT

Anatomic Considerations   49

Contractions of the Cecum and Ascending
Colon   50

Contractions of the Descending and Sigmoid
Colon   51

Motility of the Rectum and Anal Canal   52

Control of Motility   52

Clinical Significance   53

Clinical Tests   54

Summary   54

Key Words and Concepts   55

CHAPTER 7

SALIVARY SECRETION ... 57

LEONARD R. JOHNSON

Functions of Saliva   57

Anatomy and Innervation of the Salivary
Glands   58

Composition of Saliva   59
    Inorganic Composition   59
    Organic Composition   63

Regulation of Salivary Secretion   63

Summary   65

Key Words and Concepts   65

CHAPTER 8

GASTRIC SECRETION ... 67

LEONARD R. JOHNSON

Functional Anatomy   67

Secretion of Acid   70

Origin of the Electrical Potential
Difference   71

Electrolytes of Gastric Juice   71

Stimulants of Acid Secretion   72
    Role of Histamine in Acid Secretion   72

Stimulation of Acid Secretion   74
    Cephalic Phase   74
    Gastric Phase   74
    Release of Gastrin   76
    Intestinal Phase   76

Inhibition of Acid Secretion   77

Pepsin   78

Mucus   79

Intrinsic Factor   79

Growth of the Mucosa   80

Pathophysiology   80

Summary   83

Key Words and Concepts   83

Expulsion of Bile and Transport to the
Intestine   104

Clinical Applications   105

Clinical Tests   105

Summary   106

Key Words and Concepts   106

CHAPTER **9**

PANCREATIC SECRETION 85

LEONARD R. JOHNSON

Functional Anatomy   85

Mechanisms of Fluid and Electrolyte
Secretion   85

Mechanisms of Enzyme Secretion   88

Regulation of Secretion   89

Cephalic Phase   89

Gastric Phase   89

Intestinal Phase   89

Cellular Basis for Potentiation   92

Response to a Meal   93

Clinical Applications   94

Summary   94

Key Words and Concepts   95

CHAPTER **10**

BILE SECRETION AND GALLBLADDER FUNCTION . . . 97

NORMAN W. WEISBRODT

Bile Formation   97

Constituents of Bile   97

Bile Secretion   99

Bile Transport to and Storage in the
Gallbladder   102

CHAPTER **11**

DIGESTION AND ABSORPTION 107

LEONARD R. JOHNSON

Structural-Functional Associations   107

Digestion   107

Absorption   108

Mucosal Membrane   108

Transport Processes   108

Adaptation of Digestive and Absorptive
Processes   109

Carbohydrate Assimilation   109

Principal Dietary Forms   109

Digestion   110

Absorption of Digestion Products   110

Regulation of Absorption   111

*Abnormalities in Carbohydrate
Assimilation   112*

Protein Assimilation   114

Digestion   114

Development of Pancreatitis   115

Absorption of Digestion Products   115

*Abnormalities in Protein
Assimilation   116*

Lipid Assimilation   118

Digestion   118

Absorption of Lipolytic Products   119

Intracellular Events   120

Abnormalities in Lipid Assimilation   122

Vitamins   123

Summary   124

Key Words and Concepts   125

CHAPTER 12

FLUID AND ELECTROLYTE ABSORPTION 127

LEONARD R. JOHNSON

Bidirectional Fluid Flux   127

Ionic Content of Luminal Fluid   127

Transport Routes and Processes   128

Na^+-Cl^- Transport   129

K^+ Transport   131

Mechanism for Water Absorption and Secretion   131

Intestinal Secretion   132

Ca^{++} Absorption   133

Iron Absorption   134

Summary   135

Key Words and Concepts   135

CHAPTER 13

REGULATION OF FOOD INTAKE 137

LEONARD R. JOHNSON

Appetite Control   137

The Nervous System   138

Hypothalamus   138

Enteric Nervous System and Vagus Nerve   138

The Endocrine System   139

Insulin   139

Leptin   139

The Gastrointestinal System   140

Cholecystokinin   140

Peptide YY   140

Ghrelin   140

Additional Peptides   141

Treatment of Obesity   141

Summary   142

Key Words and Concepts   142

APPENDIX: REVIEW EXAMINATION . . .143

ANSWERS 151

INDEX 153

1

REGULATION
Peptides of the Gastrointestinal Tract

LEONARD R. JOHNSON

The functions of the gastrointestinal (GI) tract are regulated by peptides, derivatives of amino acids, and a variety of mediators released from nerves. All GI hormones are peptides, but it is important to realize that not all peptides found in digestive tract mucosa are hormones. The GI tract peptides can be divided into endocrines, paracrines, and neurocrines, depending on the method by which the peptide is delivered to its target site.

Endocrines, or **hormones,** are released into the general circulation and reach all tissues (unless excluded from the brain by the blood-brain barrier). Specificity is a property of the target tissue itself. Specific receptors, which recognize and bind the hormone, are present on its target tissues and absent from others. There are five established GI hormones; in addition, some GI peptides are released from endocrine cells into the blood but have no known physiologic function. Conversely, several peptides have been isolated from mucosal tissue and have potent GI effects, but no mechanism for their physiologic release has been found. Members of these latter two groups are classified as candidate hormones.

Paracrines are released from endocrine cells and diffuse through the extracellular space to their target tissues. Their effects are limited by the short distances necessary for diffusion. Nevertheless, these agents can affect large areas of the digestive tract by virtue of the scattered and abundant distributions of the cells containing them. A paracrine agent can also act on endocrine cells. Thus a paracrine may release or inhibit the release of an endocrine substance, thereby ultimately regulating a process remote from its origin. Histamine, a derivative of the amino acid histidine, is an important regulatory agent that acts as a paracrine.

Some GI peptides are located in nerves and may act as **neurocrines** or neurotransmitters. A neurocrine is released near its target tissue and needs only to diffuse across a short synaptic gap. Neurocrines conceivably may stimulate or inhibit the release of endocrines or paracrines. **Acetylcholine** (ACh), though not a peptide, is an important neuroregulator in the GI tract. One of its actions is to stimulate acid secretion from the gastric parietal cells.

GENERAL CHARACTERISTICS

The GI tract is the largest endocrine organ in the body, and its hormones were the first to be discovered. The word *hormone* was coined by W. B. Hardy and used by Starling in 1905 to describe secretin and gastrin and to convey the concept of bloodborne chemical messengers. The GI hormones are released from the mucosa of the stomach and small intestine by nervous activity, distention, and chemical stimulation coincident with the intake of food. Released into the portal circulation, the GI hormones pass through the liver to the heart and back to the digestive system to regulate its movements, secretions, and growth. These hormones also regulate the growth of the mucosa of the stomach and small and large intestines, and the growth of the exocrine pancreas.

The GI peptides have many different types of actions. Their effects on water, electrolyte, and enzyme secretion are well known, but they also influence motility, growth, and release of other hormones, as well as intestinal absorption. Many of these actions overlap; two or more GI peptides may affect the same process in the same direction, or they may inhibit each other. Many of the demonstrated actions of these peptides are pharmacologic and do not occur under normal circumstances. This chapter is concerned primarily with the physiologic effects of the GI peptides.

The actions of the GI peptides also may vary in both degree and direction among species. The actions discussed in the remainder of this chapter are those occurring in humans.

DISCOVERY

Four steps are required to establish the existence of a GI hormone. First, a physiologic event such as a meal must be demonstrated to provide the stimulus to one part of the digestive tract that subsequently alters the activity in another part. Second, the effect must persist after all nervous connections between the two parts of the tract have been severed. Third, from the site of application of the stimulus a substance must be isolated that, when injected into the blood, mimics the effect of the stimulus. Fourth, the substance must be identified chemically, and its structure must be confirmed by synthesis.

Five GI peptides have achieved full status as hormones. They are secretin, gastrin, cholecystokinin (CCK), gastric inhibitory peptide (GIP), and motilin. There is also an extensive list of "candidate" hormones whose significance has not been established. This list includes several chemically defined peptides that have significant actions in physiology or pathology but whose hormonal status has not been proved. These are pancreatic polypeptide, neurotensin, and substance P. In addition, two known hormones, glucagon and somatostatin, have been identified in GI tract mucosa; their possible function as GI hormones is currently being investigated. Some of these peptides function physiologically as paracrines or neurocrines.

Secretin, the first hormone, was discovered in 1902 by Bayliss and Starling and was described as a substance, released from the duodenal mucosa by hydrochloric acid, that stimulated pancreatic bicarbonate and fluid secretion. Jorpes and Mutt isolated it and identified its amino acid sequence in 1966. It was synthesized by Bodanszky and coworkers later the same year.

Edkins discovered **gastrin** in 1905, stating to the Royal Society that "in the process of the absorption of digested food in the stomach a substance may be separated from the cells of the mucous membrane which, passing into the blood or lymph, later stimulates the secretory cells of the stomach to functional activity." For 43 years investigators were preoccupied by the controversy over the existence of gastrin. The debate intensified when Popielski demonstrated that histamine, a ubiquitous substance present in large quantities throughout the body (including the gastric mucosa), was a powerful gastric secretagogue. In 1938 Komarov demonstrated that gastrin was a polypeptide and was different from histamine. By 1964 Gregory and his colleagues had extracted and isolated hog gastrin; Kenner and his group synthesized it the same year. After 60 years all of the criteria for establishing the existence of a GI hormone had been satisfied.

In 1928 Ivy and Oldberg described a humoral mechanism for the stimulation of gallbladder contraction initiated by the presence of fat in the intestine. The hormone was named **cholecystokinin** after its primary action. The only controversy involving CCK was a mild one over nomenclature. In 1943 Harper and Raper described a hormone released from the small intestine that stimulated pancreatic enzyme secretion and accordingly named it *pancreozymin.* As Jorpes and Mutt carried out the purification of these two substances in 1968, it became obvious that both properties resided in the same peptide. For the sake of convenience and because it was the first action described, this hormone is called CCK.

In 1969 Brown and his coworkers described the purification of a powerful enterogastrone from intestinal mucosa. **Enterogastrone** literally means a substance from the intestine (*entero-*) that inhibits (*-one*) the stomach (*gastr-*). By 1971 this peptide had been purified, isolated, sequenced, and named **gastric inhibitory peptide** for its ability to inhibit gastric secretion. Released from the intestinal mucosa by fat and glucose, GIP also stimulates insulin release. Following proof that the release of insulin was a physiologic action of the peptide, GIP became the fourth

GI hormone. The insulinotropic effect of GIP requires elevated amounts of serum glucose. For this reason, and because it is doubtful whether the inhibitory effects of the peptide on the stomach are physiologic, it has been suggested that its name be changed to glucose-dependent insulinotropic peptide. In either case it is still referred to as GIP.

Brown and his coworkers also described the purification of **motilin** in the early 1970s. Motilin is a linear 22–amino acid peptide purified from the upper small intestine. During fasting it is released cyclically and stimulates upper GI motility. Its release is under neural control and accounts for the interdigestive migrating myoelectric complex.

CHEMISTRY

The GI hormones and some related peptides can be divided into two structurally homologous families. The first consists of gastrin (Figure 1-1) and CCK (Figure 1-2). The five carboxyl-terminal (C-terminal) amino acids are identical in these two hormones. All the biologic activity of gastrin can be reproduced by the four C-terminal amino acids. This tetrapeptide, then, is the minimum fragment of gastrin needed for strong activity and is about one-sixth as active as the whole 17–amino acid molecule. The sixth amino acid from the C-terminus of gastrin is tyrosine, which may or may not be sulfated. When sulfated, the hormone is called **gastrin II.** Both forms occur with equal frequency in nature. The amino-terminus (N-terminus) of gastrin is pyroglutamyl, and the C-terminus is phenylalamide

1		2		3		4		5		6–10		11
Pyro	—	Gly	—	Pro	—	Trp	—	Leu	—	(Glu)5	—	Ala —

12		13		14		15		16		17
Tyr	—	Gly	Trp—	Met	—	Asp	—	Phe	—	NH$_2$
R										

Minimal fragment for strong activity

Gastrin I, R = H   Pyro = pyroglutamyl
Gastrin II, R = SO$_3$H

FIGURE 1-1 ■ Structure of human little gastrin (G 17).

1	2	3	4	5	6	7	8	9
Lys —	Ala —	Pro —	Ser —	Gly —	Arg —	Val —	Ser —	Met —

10	11	12	13	14	15	16	17	18
Ile —	Lys —	Asn —	Leu —	Gln —	Ser —	Leu —	Asp —	Pro —

19	20	21	22	23	24	25	26
Ser —	His —	Arg —	Ile —	Ser —	Asp —	Arg —	Asp —

27	28	29	30	31	32	33
Tyr —	Met	Gly —	Trp—	Met—	Asp—	Phe— NH$_2$
SO$_3$H		Identical to gastrin				

Minimal fragment for CCK pattern of activity

FIGURE 1-2 ■ Structure of porcine cholecystokinin (CCK)

(see Figure 1-1). Note that the NH$_2$ group following Phe does not signify that this is the N-terminus; rather, it indicates that this C-terminal amino acid is amidated. These alterations in structure protect the molecules from aminopeptidases and carboxypeptidases and allow most of them to pass through the liver without being inactivated.

Gastrin is first synthesized as a large, biologically inactive precursor called progastrin. A glycine-extended (**G-Gly**) form of gastrin is then formed by endoproteolytic processing within the G cells. G-Gly is the substrate for an amidation reaction that results in the formation of the mature, amidated gastrin. The C-terminal amide moiety is required for full biologic activity mediated by gastrin/**CCK-B** receptors. G-Gly does not stimulate the gastrin/CCK-B receptors but activates its own receptor, leading to the activation of Jun kinase and trophic effects.

CCK, which has 33 amino acids, contains a sulfated tyrosyl residue in position 7 from the C-terminus (see Figure 1-2). CCK can activate gastrin receptors (e.g., those for acid secretion, also called CCK-B receptors); gastrin can activate CCK receptors (e.g., those for gallbladder contraction, also called CCK-A receptors). Each hormone, however, is much more potent at its own receptors than at those of its homologue. CCK is always sulfated in nature, and desulfation produces a peptide with the gastrin pattern of activity. The minimally active fragment for the CCK pattern of activity is therefore the C-terminal heptapeptide. In summary, peptides belonging to the gastrin/CCK family having a tyrosyl residue in position 6 from the C-terminus or an unsulfated one in position 7 possess the gastrin pattern of activity—strong stimulation of gastric acid secretion and weak contraction of the gallbladder. Peptides with a sulfated tyrosyl residue in position 7 have cholecystokinetic potency and are weak stimulators of gastric acid secretion. Obviously the tetrapeptide itself and all fragments less than 7 amino acids long possess gastrin-like activity.

The second group of peptides is homologous to secretin and includes **vasoactive intestinal peptide** (VIP), GIP, and **glucagon,** in addition to secretin (Figure 1-3). Secretin has 27 amino acids, all of which are required for substantial activity. Pancreatic glucagon has 29 amino acids, 14 of which are identical to those of secretin. Glucagon-like immunoreactivity has been isolated from the small intestine, but the physiologic significance of this **enteroglucagon** has not been established. Glucagon has no active fragment, and like secretin the whole molecule is required before any activity is observed. There is evidence that secretin exists as a helix; thus the entire amino acid sequence may be necessary to form a tertiary structure with biologic activity.

GIP and VIP each have 9 amino acids that are identical to those of secretin. Each has many of the same actions as those of secretin and glucagon. This group

of peptides is discussed in greater detail later in the chapter.

Most peptide hormones are heterogeneous and occur in two or more molecular forms. Gastrin, secretin, and CCK all have been shown to exist in more than one form. Gastrin was originally isolated from hog antral mucosa as a heptadecapeptide (see Figure 1-1), which is now referred to as little gastrin (G 17). It accounts for 90% of antral gastrin. Yalow and Berson demonstrated heterogeneity by showing that the major component of gastrin immunoactivity in the serum was a larger molecule that they called big gastrin. On isolation, big gastrin was found to contain 34 amino acids; hence it is called G 34. Trypsin splits G 34 to yield G 17 plus a heptadecapeptide different from G 17. Therefore, G 34 is not simply a dimer of G 17. An additional gastrin molecule (G 14) has been isolated from tissue and contains the C-terminal tetradecapeptide of gastrin. Current evidence indicates that most G 17 is produced from pro G 17 and most G 34 from pro G 34. Thus G 34 is not a necessary intermediate in the production of G 17.

During the interdigestive (basal) state, most human serum gastrin is G 34. Unlike those of other species, the duodenal mucosa of humans contains significant amounts of gastrin. This is primarily G 34 and is released in small amounts during the basal state. After a meal a large quantity of antral gastrin, primarily G 17, is released and provides most of the stimulus for

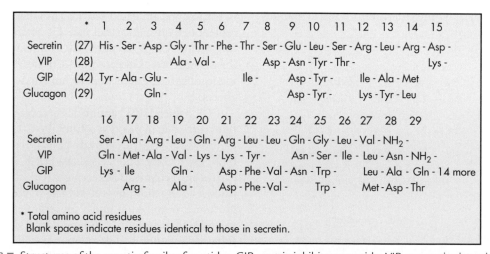

	*	1	2	3	4	5	6	7	8	9	10	11	12	13	14	15
Secretin	(27)	His	Ser	Asp	Gly	Thr	Phe	Thr	Ser	Glu	Leu	Ser	Arg	Leu	Arg	Asp -
VIP	(28)				Ala	Val				Asp	Asn	Tyr	Thr			Lys -
GIP	(42)	Tyr	Ala	Glu				Ile		Asp	Tyr		Ile	Ala	Met	
Glucagon	(29)			Gln						Asp	Tyr		Lys	Tyr	Leu	

	16	17	18	19	20	21	22	23	24	25	26	27	28	29
Secretin	Ser	Ala	Arg	Leu	Gln	Arg	Leu	Leu	Gln	Gly	Leu	Val - NH_2		
VIP	Gln	Met	Ala	Val	Lys	Lys	Tyr		Asn	Ser	Ile	Leu	Asn - NH_2	
GIP	Lys	Ile		Gln		Asp	Phe	Val	Asn	Trp		Leu	Ala	Gln - 14 more
Glucagon		Arg		Ala		Asp	Phe	Val		Trp		Met	Asp	Thr

* Total amino acid residues
Blank spaces indicate residues identical to those in secretin.

FIGURE 1-3 ■ Structures of the secretin family of peptides. GIP, gastric inhibitory peptide; VIP, vasoactive intestinal peptide.

gastric acid secretion. Smaller amounts of G 34 are released from both the antral and the duodenal mucosa. G 17 and G 34 are equipotent, although the half-life of G 34 is 38 minutes and that of G 17 is about 7 minutes.

DISTRIBUTION AND RELEASE

The GI hormones are located in endocrine cells scattered throughout the GI mucosa from the stomach through the colon. The cells containing individual hormones are not clumped together but are dispersed among the epithelial cells. The nature of this distribution makes it virtually impossible to surgically remove the source of one of the GI hormones and examine the effect of its absence without compromising the digestive function of the animal.

The endocrine cells of the gut are members of a widely distributed system termed **amine precursor uptake decarboxylation** (APUD) cells. These cells all are derived from neuroendocrine-programmed cells originating in the embryonic ectoblast.

The distributions of the individual GI hormones are shown in Figure 1-4. Gastrin is most abundant in antral and duodenal mucosa. Most of its release under physiologic conditions is from the antrum. Secretin, CCK, GIP, and motilin are found in the duodenum and jejunum.

Ultrastructurally, GI endocrine cells have hormone-containing granules concentrated at their bases, close to the capillaries. The granules discharge, releasing their hormones in response to a number of events that are either the direct or the indirect result of neural, physical, and chemical stimuli associated with eating a meal and the presence of that meal within the digestive tract. These endocrine cells have microvilli on their apical

TABLE 1-1					
Releasers of Gastrointestinal Hormones					
	HORMONE				
RELEASER	*Gastrin*	*CCK*	*Secretin*	*GIP*	*Motilin*
Protein	S	S	0	S	0
Fat	0	S	S–	S	S–
Carbohydrate	0	0	0	S	0
Acid	I	S–	S	0	S–
Distention	S	0	0	0	0
Nerve	S	0	0	0	S

CCK, cholecystokinin; GIP, gastric inhibitory peptide; I, inhibits release physiologically; S, physiologic stimulus for release; S–, of secondary importance; 0, no effect.

borders that presumably contain receptors for sampling the luminal contents.

Table 1-1 lists the stimuli that are physiologically important releasers of the GI hormones. Gastrin and motilin are the only hormones demonstrated as being released directly by neural stimulation. Protein in the form of peptides and single amino acids releases both gastrin and CCK. Fatty acids containing eight or more carbon atoms or their monoglycerides are the most potent stimuli for CCK release. Fat must be broken down into an absorbable form before releasing CCK, evidence that the receptors for release are triggered during the process of absorption.

There is evidence for intestinal releasing factors that are secreted into the intestine of a number of species, including humans, that stimulate the release of CCK. Pancreatic enzymes inactivate these releasing factors. The ingestion and presence of a meal in the intestine result in temporary binding of trypsin and other

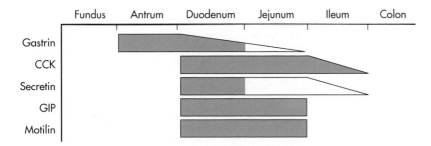

FIGURE 1-4 ■ Distribution of the gastrointestinal hormones. *Shaded areas* indicate where the most release occurs under normal conditions. CCK, cholecystokinin; GIP, gastric inhibitory peptide.

proteases, allowing the releasing factors to remain active and stimulate CCK secretion. Thus, this mechanism acts as a negative feedback control on pancreatic enzyme secretion.

Carbohydrate, the remaining major foodstuff, does not alter the release of gastrin, secretin, or CCK to a significant extent but does stimulate GIP release. GIP also is released by fat and protein. The strongest stimulus for secretin release is H^+. Secretin is released when the pH in the duodenum falls below 4.5. Secretin also is released by fatty acids. This may be a significant mechanism for secretin release because the concentration of fatty acids in the lumen is often high. CCK can also be released by acid, but except during hypersecretion of acid, the physiologic significance of this mechanism of release has not been established. The purely physical stimulus of distention activates antral receptors, causing gastrin release; for example, inflating a balloon in the antrum releases gastrin. During a meal the pressure of ingested food initiates this response. The magnitude of the response is not as great as originally believed, however, and the contribution that distention makes to the total amount of gastrin released in humans probably is minor. Gastrin also can be released by calcium, decaffeinated coffee, and wine. Pure alcohol in the same concentration as that of wine does not release gastrin but does stimulate acid secretion. Motilin is released cyclically (approximately every 90 minutes) during fasting. This release is prevented by atropine and ingestion of a mixed meal. Acid and fat in the duodenum, however, increase motilin release.

In addition to releasing secretin, acid exerts an important negative feedback control of gastrin release. Acidification of the antral mucosa below a pH of 3.5 inhibits gastrin release. Patients with atrophic gastritis, pernicious anemia, or other conditions characterized by the chronic decrease of acid-secreting cells and hyposecretion of acid may have extremely high serum concentrations of gastrin because of the absence of this inhibitory mechanism.

There are several instances in which hormones alter the release of GI peptides. Secretin and glucagon, for example, both inhibit gastrin release. CCK has been shown to stimulate glucagon release, and four GI hormones (secretin, gastrin, CCK, and GIP) increase insulin secretion. Elevated serum calcium stimulates both gastrin and CCK release. It is doubtful whether any of these

mechanisms, with the exception of release of insulin by GIP, play a role in normal GI physiology. Some, however, may become important when circulating levels of hormones or calcium are altered by disease.

ACTIONS AND INTERACTIONS

The effects of pure GI hormones have been tested on almost every secretory, motor, and absorptive function of the GI tract. Each peptide has some action on almost every target tested. Even though large doses of hormone sometimes are necessary to produce an effect, either stimulatory or inhibitory, it indicates that receptors for each hormone are present on most target tissues. The myriad activities possessed by these peptides are summarized in Table 1-2.

The important physiologic actions of the GI hormones are depicted in Table 1-3. Numerous guidelines have been proposed for determining whether an action is physiologic. The action should occur in response to endogenous hormone released by normal stimuli (i.e., those present during a meal). In other words, an exogenous dose of hormone should produce the effect in question without elevating serum hormone levels above those produced by a meal. An acceptable guideline for

TABLE 1-2
Actions of Gastrointestinal Hormones

ACTION	HORMONE				
	Gastrin	CCK	Secretin	GIP	Motilin
Acid secretion	S	S	I	I	
Gastric emptying	I	I	I	I	
Pancreatic HCO_3^- secretion	S	S	S	0	
Pancreatic HCO_3^- enzyme secretion	S	S	S	0	
Bile HCO_3^- secretion	S	S	S	0	
Gallbladder contraction	S	S	S		
Gastric motility	S	S	I	I	S
Intestinal motility	S	S	I		S
Insulin release	S	S	S	S	
Mucosal growth	S	S	I		
Pancreatic growth	S	S	S		

CCK, cholecystokinin; GIP, gastric inhibitory peptide; I, inhibits; S, stimulates; 0, no effect; *blank spaces*, not yet tested.

TABLE 1-3

Important Actions of Gastrointestinal Hormones

ACTION	HORMONE				
	Gastrin	*CCK*	*Secretin*	*GIP*	*Motilin*
Acid secretion	S		I	I	
Pancreatic HCO$_3^-$ secretion		S	S		
Pancreatic enzyme secretion		S			
Bile HCO$_3^-$ secretion			S		
Gallbladder contraction		S			
Gastric emptying	I				
Insulin release				S	
Mucosal growth	S				
Pancreatic growth		S	S		
Gastric motility					S
Intestinal motility					S

CCK, cholecystokinin; GIP, gastric inhibitory peptide; I, inhibits; S, stimulates.

exogenous infusion is a dose that produces 50% of the maximal response (D_{50}) of the primary action of the hormone. The hormone should be administered as a continuous intravenous infusion rather than as a single bolus because the latter produces transient, unphysiologically high serum levels.

The primary action of gastrin is the stimulation of gastric acid secretion. It does this by causing the release of histamine (a potent acid secretagogue) from the **enterochromaffin-like** (ECL) **cells** of the stomach and by direct action on the parietal cells. Gastrin is the most important regulator of gastric acid secretion. There is considerable debate on the role of gastrin in regulating the tone of the lower esophageal sphincter, with the bulk of the evidence indicating no normal role for gastrin in regulation.

One of the most important and recently discovered actions of GI hormones is their trophic activity. Gastrin stimulates synthesis of ribonucleic acid (RNA), protein, and deoxyribonucleic acid (DNA), as well as growth of the mucosa of the small intestine, colon, and oxyntic gland area of the stomach. If most endogenous gastrin is removed by antrectomy, these tissues atrophy. Exogenous gastrin prevents the atrophy. Patients with tumors that constantly secrete gastrin exhibit hyperplasia

and hypertrophy of the acid-secreting portion of the stomach. Gastrin also stimulates the growth of ECL cells. Continued hypersecretion of gastrin results in ECL cell hyperplasia, which may develop into carcinoid tumors. The trophic effects of gastrin are restricted to GI tissues and are counteracted by secretin. The trophic action of gastrin is a direct effect that can be demonstrated in tissue culture.

As mentioned previously, G-Gly also has trophic effects. G-Gly is far less potent (by at least four orders of magnitude) than gastrin in stimulating gastric acid secretion. However, G-Gly is stored in gut tissues, is secreted with gastrin from antral G cells, and reaches concentrations in plasma equal to those of gastrin. Although antagonists of the CCK-B/gastrin receptor block the trophic effects of gastrin, they have no effect on the growth-promoting actions of G-Gly. Additional evidence suggests that the growth-related receptors for G-Gly work in concert with gastrin to regulate the functional development of the gut.

The primary effect of secretin is the stimulation of pancreatic fluid and bicarbonate secretion; one of the primary actions of CCK is the stimulation of pancreatic enzyme secretion. In addition, CCK has a physiologically important interaction in potentiating the primary effect of secretin. Thus CCK greatly increases the pancreatic bicarbonate response to low circulating levels of secretin.

Both CCK and secretin also stimulate the growth of the exocrine pancreas. CCK exerts a stronger effect than secretin, but the combination of the two hormones produces a potentiated response in rats that is truly remarkable. It is likely that the effects of these two hormones on pancreatic growth are as important as their effects on pancreatic secretion.

In addition to its effects on the pancreas, secretin stimulates biliary secretion of fluid and bicarbonate. This action is shared by CCK, but secretin is the most potent choleretic of the GI hormones. In dogs, secretin is a potent inhibitor of gastrin-stimulated acid secretion. This action, however, is probably not physiologically important in humans. The ability of secretin to inhibit acid secretion may be important in some human diseases, however, and students should be aware of this action. Secretin has been nicknamed "nature's antacid" because almost all of its actions reduce the amount of acid in the duodenum. The only known exception to this statement is secretin's pepsigogic activity. Secretin is second only to ACh in promoting pepsinogen secretion from the chief cells of the stomach. Under normal circumstances only small amounts of secretin are released, making it doubtful whether secretin stimulates pepsin secretion physiologically.

In addition to its physiologic actions on pancreatic and biliary secretion, CCK regulates gallbladder contraction and gastric emptying. Of the GI peptides, CCK is the most potent regulator of gallbladder contraction; it is approximately 100 times more effective than the gastrin tetrapeptide in contracting the gallbladder. CCK causes significant inhibition of gastric emptying in doses equal to the D_{50} of pancreatic secretion. Gastrin also inhibits gastric emptying, but the effective dose is about 6 times the D_{50} for stimulation of acid secretion by gastrin. These data support conclusions that CCK physiologically inhibits gastric emptying and gastrin does not.

There are several peptides, including secretin and GIP, that are enterogastrones. GIP was originally discovered because of its ability to inhibit gastric acid secretion and may well have been the original enterogastrone described by Ivy and Farrell in 1925. Its action has not been established as physiologically significant in the innervated stomach. GIP, however, is a strong stimulator of insulin release and is responsible for the fact that an oral glucose load releases more insulin and is metabolized more rapidly than an equal amount of glucose administered intravenously.

Motilin stimulates the so-called *migrating motility* or *myoelectric complex* that moves through the stomach and small bowel every 90 minutes in the fasted GI tract. Its cyclical release into the blood is inhibited by the ingestion of a meal. This is the only known function of this peptide.

CANDIDATE HORMONES

Earlier in this chapter, certain peptides isolated from digestive tract tissue were mentioned that may, at a later date, qualify as hormones. These often are referred to as *candidate*, or *putative*, *hormones*. Many have been proposed, but interest is greatest for those listed in Table 1-4. Enteroglucagon belongs to the secretin family. **Pancreatic polypeptide** and **peptide YY** (tyrosine-tyrosine) belong to a separate family and are unrelated to either gastrin or secretin.

TABLE 1-4
Candidate Hormones

PEPTIDE	RELEASED BY	ACTION(S)
Pancreatic polypeptide	Protein Fat Glucose	↓Pancreatic HCO_3^- and enzyme secretion
Peptide YY	Fat	↓Gastric secretion ↓Gastric emptying
Enteroglucagon	Hexose Fat	↓Gastric secretion ↓Gastric emptying ↑Insulin release

↓, inhibits; ↑, stimulates.

Pancreatic polypeptide was first identified as a minor impurity in insulin. It was then isolated and found to be a linear peptide with 36 amino acid residues. From a physiologic viewpoint the most important action of pancreatic polypeptide is the inhibition of both pancreatic bicarbonate and enzyme secretion, because this effect has the lowest dose requirement. Most constituents of a meal release pancreatic polypeptide, and the serum levels reached are sufficient to inhibit pancreatic secretion. Because the peak rate of pancreatic secretion during a meal is less than the maximal rate that can be achieved with exogenous stimuli, it is possible that pancreatic polypeptide modulates this response under normal conditions. Before it can be concluded that pancreatic polypeptide is responsible for the physiologic inhibition of pancreatic secretion, it must be shown that this actually occurs and that pancreatic polypeptide is the agent involved. The fact that the peptide is located in the pancreas and cannot be removed without also removing its target organ makes this evidence difficult to obtain.

Peptide YY was discovered in porcine small intestine and named for its N-terminal and C-terminal amino acid residues—both tyrosines. Of its 36 amino acid residues, 18 are identical to those of pancreatic polypeptide. Peptide YY is released by meals, especially by fat. It may appear in plasma in concentrations sufficient to inhibit gastric secretion and emptying and thus qualify as an enterogastrone. Its effects do not appear to be direct in that it does not inhibit secretion in response to gastrin or histamine. It does inhibit neurally stimulated secretion, but its final status as an enterogastrone has not been determined. Peptide YY also inhibits intestinal motility, and this effect is believed by some investigators to enhance luminal nutrient digestion and absorption.

The enteroglucagons are products of the same gene processed in the pancreatic alpha cell to form glucagon. The intestinal L cell makes three forms of glucagon, one of which, **glucagon-like peptide-1** (GLP-1), may have important physiologic actions. This 30–amino acid peptide is a potent insulin releaser, even in the absence of hyperglycemia, and also inhibits gastric secretion and emptying. GLP-1 may mediate the so-called ileal brake—the inhibition of gastric and pancreatic secretion and motility that occurs when lipids and/or carbohydrates are infused into the ileum in amounts sufficient to cause malabsorption.

NEUROCRINES

Originally all GI peptides were believed to originate from endocrine cells and therefore be either hormones or candidate hormones. With the advent of sophisticated immunocytochemical techniques for tissue localization of peptides, it became apparent that many were contained within the nerves of the gut.

Numerous peptides have been found in both the brain and the digestive tract mucosa. The first of these to be isolated was substance P, which in the GI tract has the property of stimulating intestinal motility and gallbladder contraction. The only other peptide isolated from both the brain and gut and known to have an identical structure in both sites is neurotensin. Neurotensin increases blood glucose by stimulating glycogenolysis and glucagon release and inhibiting insulin release. Other peptides have been isolated from one site and identified by radioimmunoassay in the other. These include motilin, CCK, and VIP, which were first isolated from the gut. Enkephalin, somatostatin, and thyrotropin-releasing factor were first isolated from the brain and later found in the gut. Gastrin, VIP, somatostatin, and enkephalin also are present in the nerves of the gut.

There are three peptides that function physiologically in the gut as neurocrines (listed in Table 1-5). Originally investigators thought VIP was found in gut endocrine cells. It is now known to be localized within the gut exclusively within nerves. It physiologically mediates

TABLE 1-5		
Neurocrines		
PEPTIDE	**LOCATION**	**ACTION**
VIP	Mucosa and muscle of gut	Relaxation of gut smooth muscle
GRP or bombesin	Gastric mucosa	↑Gastrin release
Enkephalins	Mucosa and muscle of gut	↑Smooth muscle tone

GRP, gastrin-releasing peptide; VIP, vasoactive intestinal peptide; ↑, stimulates.

the relaxation of GI smooth muscle. Smooth muscle is innervated by VIP-containing fibers, and VIP is released during relaxation. VIP relaxes smooth muscle, and VIP antiserum blocks neurally induced relaxation. In addition, there is strong evidence that VIP physiologically mediates relaxation of smooth muscle in blood vessels and thus may be responsible for vasodilation. Besides these effects, VIP has many of the actions of its relatives, secretin and GIP, when injected into the bloodstream. It stimulates pancreatic secretion, inhibits gastric secretion, and stimulates intestinal secretion. Many of the effects of VIP on smooth muscle are mediated by nitric oxide (NO); VIP stimulates the synthesis of this potent smooth muscle relaxant.

Numerous biologically active peptides have been isolated from amphibian skin and later found to have mammalian counterparts. One of these, called *bombesin* after the species of frog from which it was isolated, is a potent releaser of gastrin. The mammalian counterpart of bombesin is gastrin-releasing peptide (GRP), which has been found in the nerves of the gastric mucosa. GRP is released by vagal stimulation and mediates the vagal release of gastrin. Luminal protein digestion products may also stimulate gastrin release through a GRP-mediated mechanism.

Two pentapeptides isolated from pig and calf brains activate opiate receptors and are called *enkephalins*. They are identical except that the C-terminal amino acid is methionine in one and leucine in the other. These compounds are present in nerves within both the smooth muscle and the mucosa of the GI tract. Opiate receptors on circular smooth muscle cells mediate contraction, and leuenkephalin and metenkephalin cause contraction of the lower esophageal, pyloric, and ileocecal sphincters. The enkephalins function physiologically at these sites and also may be an intricate part of the peristaltic mechanism. The effect of opiates on intestinal motility is to slow transit of material through the gut. These peptides also inhibit intestinal secretion. The combination of these actions probably accounts for the effectiveness of opiates in treating diarrhea.

Absent from Table 1-5 is pituitary adenylate cyclase–activating peptide (PACAP), the newest member of the secretin family. If somatostatin is blocked, injection of PACAP stimulates the release of histamine from ECL cells and, therefore, stimulates acid secretion. PACAP also stimulates ECL cell growth, so its actions are similar to those of gastrin. It may be a significant neural mediator of ECL cell function, but direct evidence that ECL cells are innervated by PACAP-containing fibers is missing.

PARACRINES

Paracrines are like hormones in that they are released from endocrine cells. They are similar to neurocrines because they interact with receptors close to the point of their release. The biologic significance of an endocrine can be assessed by correlating physiologic events with changes in blood levels of the hormone in question. Because the area of release of both paracrines and neurocrines is restricted, there are no comparable methods for proving the biologic significance of one of these agents. Current experiments examine the effects of specific pharmacologic blockers or antisera directed toward these substances. In vitro perfused organs are also useful in examining paracrine mediators. These systems allow an investigator to collect and assay small volumes of venous perfusate for the agent in question.

One GI peptide, **somatostatin,** functions physiologically as a paracrine to inhibit gastrin release and gastric acid secretion. Somatostatin was first isolated from the hypothalamus as a growth hormone release–inhibitory factor. It has since been shown to exist throughout the gastric and duodenal mucosa and the pancreas in high concentrations and inhibit the release of all gut hormones. Somatostatin mediates the inhibition of gastrin release occurring when the antral mucosa is acidified. Somatostatin also directly inhibits acid secretion from the parietal cells. These are important physiologic actions of this peptide.

Histamine is a second important paracrine agent. Produced in ECL cells by the decarboxylation of histidine, histamine is released by gastrin and then stimulates acid secretion from the gastric parietal cells. Histamine also potentiates the action of gastrin and ACh on acid secretion. This is why the histamine H_2 receptor–blocking drugs, such as cimetidine (Tagamet) and ranitidine (Zantac), are effective inhibitors of acid secretion regardless of the stimulus.

CLINICAL APPLICATIONS

Non–beta cell tumors of the pancreas or duodenal tumors may produce gastrin and continually release it into the blood. This disease is known as *gastrinoma* or *Zollinger-Ellison syndrome*. The tumors are small and difficult to define and resect; if metastasizing, they grow slowly. Gastrin is released from these tumors at a high spontaneous rate that is not altered by feeding. The hypergastrinemia results in hypersecretion of gastric acid through two mechanisms. First, the trophic action of gastrin leads to increased parietal cell mass and acid secretory capacity. Second, increased serum gastrin levels constantly stimulate secretion from the hyperplastic mucosa. The complications of this disease—fulminant peptic ulceration, diarrhea, steatorrhea, and hypokalemia—are caused by the presence of large amounts of acid in the small bowel. The continual presence of acid in the duodenum overwhelms the neutralizing ability of the pancreas, erodes the mucosa, and produces ulcers. In large amounts gastrin inhibits absorption of fluid and electrolytes by the intestine, thereby adding to the large volumes of fluid (up to 10 liters [L]/day) entering the intestine. Increased intestinal transit probably also contributes to the diarrhea. Steatorrhea is produced by inactivation of pancreatic lipase and precipitation of bile salts at a low luminal pH. Because the tumors are difficult to resect and the clinical manifestations are caused by hypersecretion of gastric acid, the preferred surgical treatment is removal of the target organ (the stomach). Although gastrin levels remain elevated, total gastrectomy stops the ulceration and diarrhea. This disease also may be treated nonsurgically with some of the powerful new drugs that inhibit acid secretion (see Chapter 8).

The only other clinical condition attributed to the overproduction of a GI peptide concerns VIP. Pancreatic cholera, or watery diarrhea syndrome, is a frequently lethal disease resulting from the secretion of a peptide by a pancreatic islet cell tumor. This peptide is a potent stimulus for intestinal secretion of the fluid and electrolytes that produce the copious diarrhea. VIP has been identified in both the tumor tissue and the serum of these patients. Its ability to stimulate cholera-like fluid secretion from the intestine indicates that it is responsible for this disease.

CLINICAL TESTS

Gastrin is routinely measured by radioimmunoassay in clinical laboratories. Normal serum gastrin values must be set by each laboratory for its particular assay. If the normal mean serum gastrin concentration is taken as 50 picograms (pg)/milliliter (mL), serum gastrin in fasting patients with gastrinoma usually exceeds 200 pg/mL. The degree of overlap between patients with gastrinoma and those with ordinary duodenal ulcer disease means that specific tests are required to diagnose the gastrinoma.

The tests most widely used in the evaluation of hypergastrinemia include stimulation with protein meals, intravenous calcium infusion, and secretin infusion. Patients with Zollinger-Ellison syndrome may not release gastrin in detectable amounts in response to food. This may be due to the low pH of gastric contents, which is caused by ongoing acid secretion stimulated by preexisting high serum gastrin levels. Acid in the antrum inhibits gastrin release, and any gastrin that might be released would be difficult to detect against the already high serum levels.

Gastrinoma patients may have an exaggerated acid secretory response to calcium infusions caused by the release of gastrin from tumor tissue. This test is run by infusing 5 milligrams (mg) of ionizable calcium per kg per hour as calcium gluconate for 3 hours while simultaneously measuring acid secretion and collecting blood samples at hourly intervals for gastrin determination. Peak gastrin responses are usually obtained 3 hours after calcium infusion is begun. In most patients with gastrinoma, serum gastrin concentrations will at least double so that the gastrin values will be over 500 pg/mL. Patients with ordinary ulcer disease may show moderate increases in serum gastrin with calcium infusion, but absolute gastrin values after stimulation seldom exceed 200 to 300 pg/mL.

The most specific and easiest test to administer for gastrinoma is secretin injection. Secretin inhibits antral gastrin release, yet it stimulates tumor gastrin release in almost all patients with gastrinoma. Secretin (1 unit [U]/kg) is given as a rapid intravenous injection and causes a peak increase in serum gastrin 5 to 10 minutes later. In a patient with definitely increased basal serum gastrin and acid hypersecretion, a doubling of serum gastrin at 5 to 10 minutes strongly indicates the presence of a gastrinoma.

SUMMARY

1. The functions of the GI tract are regulated by mediators acting as hormones (endocrines), paracrines, or neurocrines.
2. Two chemically related families of peptides are responsible for much of the regulation of GI function. These are gastrin/CCK peptides and a second group containing secretin, VIP, GIP, and glucagon.
3. The GI hormones are located in endocrine cells scattered throughout the mucosa and released by chemicals in food, neural activity, or physical distention.
4. The GI peptides have many pharmacologic actions, but only a few of these are physiologically significant.
5. Gastrin, CCK, secretin, GIP, and motilin are important GI hormones.
6. Somatostatin and histamine have important functions as paracrine agents.
7. VIP, bombesin (or GRP), and the enkephalins are released from nerves and mediate many important functions of the digestive tract.

KEY WORDS AND CONCEPTS

- Endocrines/hormones
- Paracrines
- Neurocrines
- Acetylcholine
- Secretin
- Gastrin

- Cholecystokinin
- Enterogastrone
- Gastric inhibitory peptide
- Motilin
- Gastrin II
- Vasoactive intestinal peptide
- Glucagon
- Enteroglucagon
- G-Gly
- CCK-B receptor
- Amine precursor uptake decarboxylation
- Enterochromaffin-like cells
- Pancreatic polypeptide
- Peptide YY
- Glucagon-like peptide-1
- Somatostatin
- Histamine

REFERENCES

Dockray GJ: Physiology of enteric neuropeptides. In Johnson LR (ed): Physiology of the Gastrointestinal Tract, 3rd ed. New York, Raven Press, 1994.

Johnson LR: Regulation of gastrointestinal mucosal growth. In Johnson LR (ed): Physiology of the Gastrointestinal Tract, 3rd ed. New York, Raven Press, 1994.

Makhlouf GM (ed): Handbook of Physiology, Section 6: The Gastrointestinal System, vol 2: Neural and Endocrine Biology. Bethesda, MD, American Physiological Society, 1989.

Modlin IM, Sachs G: Acid Related Diseases. Milan, Schnetztor Verlag Gmbh D-Konstanz, 1998.

Pearse AGE, Takor T: Embryology of the diffuse neuroendocrine system and its relationship to the common peptides. Fed Proc 38: 2288-2294, 1979.

Rozengurt E, Walsh JH: Gastrin, CCK, signaling, and cancer. Annu Rev Physiol 63:49-76, 2001.

Solcia E, Capella C, Buffa R, et al: Endocrine cells of the digestive system. In Johnson LR (ed): Physiology of the Gastrointestinal Tract, 2nd ed. New York, Raven Press, 1987.

Walsh JH: Gastrointestinal hormones. In Johnson LR (ed): Physiology of the Gastrointestinal Tract, 3rd ed. New York, Raven Press, 1994.

Walsh JH, Grossman MI: Gastrin. N Engl J Med 292:1324-1332, 1337-1384, 1975.

Walsh JH, Grossman MI: The Zollinger-Ellison syndrome. Gastroenterology 65:140-165, 1973.

2

REGULATION
Nerves and Smooth Muscle

NORMAN W. WEISBRODT

S ecretory, motility, and absorptive functions of the gastrointestinal (GI) system must be integrated to accomplish digestion and absorption of meals and maintain homeostasis between meals. This integration is mediated by regulatory systems that monitor events within the body (primarily the GI tract) and in the external environment. The information is then processed such that appropriate commands to increase or decrease activities of the various organs are given. In all known cases, these commands are mediated through the actions of specific chemicals on target cells of the digestive organs. The manner in which these chemicals reach the target cells defines the various regulatory systems. In Chapter 1, the endocrine, paracrine, and neurocrine systems were discussed. In this chapter, the role of the nervous (neurocrine) system is considered in more detail.

Although the regulatory systems act to integrate the activities of the GI system, most secretory, absorptive, and muscle cells possess intrinsic activities that give them a degree of autonomy. Thus function arises out of the interaction of regulatory systems and local intrinsic properties. The basic properties and intrinsic activities of each type of secretory and absorptive cell are discussed in separate chapters that deal with the secretion and absorption of specific chemicals. The basic properties and intrinsic activities of the smooth muscle cells are discussed in this chapter.

ANATOMY OF THE AUTONOMIC NERVOUS SYSTEM

The GI tract is innervated by the **autonomic nervous system** (ANS). It is called the ANS because people normally are neither conscious of its activities nor exerting any willful control over them. The ANS can be divided into the extrinsic nervous system and the intrinsic, or enteric, nervous system.

The **extrinsic nervous system** is in turn divided into parasympathetic and sympathetic branches (Figure 2-1). **Parasympathetic innervation** is supplied primarily by the vagus and pelvic nerves. Long preganglionic axons arise from cell bodies within the medulla of the brain and the sacral region of the spinal cord. These preganglionic nerves enter the various organs of the GI tract, where they synapse mainly with cells of the enteric nervous system. In addition, these same nerve bundles contain many afferent nerves whose receptors lie within the various tissues of the gut. These nerves project to the brain and spinal cord to provide sensory input for integration.

Sympathetic innervation is supplied by nerves that run between the spinal cord and the prevertebral ganglia and between these ganglia and the organs of the gut. Preganglionic efferent fibers arise within the cord and end in the prevertebral ganglia. Postganglionic fibers from these ganglia then innervate primarily the elements of the enteric nervous system. Few fibers end directly on secretory, absorptive, or muscle cells. Afferent fibers

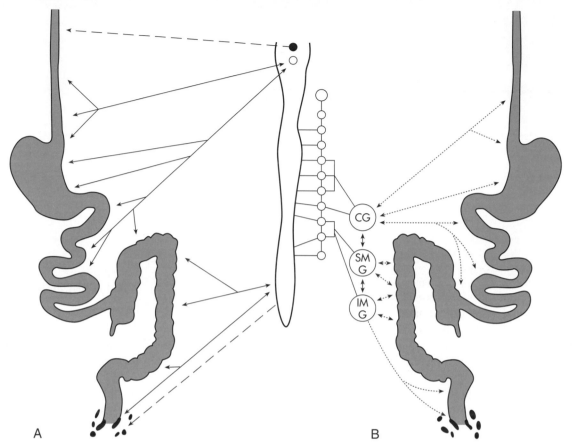

FIGURE 2-1 ■ Extrinsic branches of the autonomic nervous system. **A,** Parasympathetic. *Dashed lines* indicate the cholinergic innervation of striated muscle in the esophagus and external anal sphincter. *Solid lines* indicate the afferent and preganglionic efferent innervation of the rest of the gastrointestinal tract. **B,** Sympathetic. *Solid lines* denote the afferent and preganglionic efferent connections between the spinal cord and the prevertebral ganglia. *Dashed lines* indicate the afferent and postganglionic efferent innervation. CG, celiac ganglion; IMG, inferior mesenteric ganglion; SMG, superior mesenteric ganglion.

also are present within the sympathetic division. These nerves project back to the prevertebral ganglia and/or the spinal cord. Thus an abundance of sensory information also is available via these nerves.

Elements of the **intrinsic,** or **enteric, nervous system** are grouped into several anatomically distinct networks, of which the **myenteric** and **submucosal plexuses** are the most prominent. These plexuses consist of nerve cell bodies, axons, dendrites, and nerve endings. Processes from the neurons of the plexuses do not just innervate target cells such as smooth muscle, secretory cells, and absorptive cells. They also connect to sensory receptors and interdigitate with processes from other neurons located both inside and outside the plexus. Thus, pathways within the enteric nervous system can be multisynaptic, and integration of activities can take place entirely within the enteric nervous system (Figure 2-2), as well as in the ganglia of the extrinsic nerves, the spinal cord, and the brainstem.

A large number of chemicals serve as **neurocrines** within the ANS. Several of these chemicals have been localized within specific pathways, and a few have defined physiologic roles. Most of the extrinsic, preganglionic, efferent fibers contain **acetylcholine** (ACh). This transmitter exerts its action on neurons contained within the prevertebral ganglia and enteric nervous system.

FIGURE 2-2 ■ Schematic of a horizontal section through the wall of the intestine at the level of the myenteric plexus, showing examples of reflex pathways depicted in a short segment of intestine. The first parts of descending inhibitory and ascending excitatory reflex pathways for propulsive reflexes are depicted. Intrinsic primary afferent neurons (IPANs) are circumferentially oriented and form self-reinforcing networks. They provide outputs to ascending and descending interneurons and monosynaptic connections to motor neurons. One type of descending interneuron (*bottom part* of diagram), which is involved in conducting the migrating myoelectric complex along the small intestine, receives few inputs from IPANs but connects with motor neurons. Some of the excitatory transmitters that have been localized to intrinsic nerves are acetylcholine and the tachykinins; some of the inhibitory transmitters are nitric oxide and vasoactive intestinal peptide. *Not shown* are the extrinsic nerves that provide synaptic input to the intrinsic nerves and sensory information to neurons in extrinsic ganglia, the spinal cord, and the brain. *(Adapted from Furness JB: The Enteric Nervous System. Blackwell, Malden, Mass, 2006.)*

Norepinephrine is found in many nerve endings of the postganglionic efferent nerves of the sympathetic nervous system. This transmitter also exerts its effects primarily on neurons of the enteric nervous system. Within the enteric nervous system, ACh, **serotonin, vasoactive intestinal peptide** (VIP), **nitric oxide** (NO), and **somatostatin** have been localized to interneurons. ACh and the tachykinins (TKs) (such as **substance P**) have been localized to nerves that are excitatory to the muscle; VIP and NO have been localized to inhibitory nerves to the muscle. In many instances, more than one transmitter can be localized to the same nerve. The goals of mapping neural circuits within the extrinsic and enteric nervous system and elucidating their functions are far from complete.

NEUROHUMORAL REGULATION OF GASTROINTESTINAL FUNCTION

Although it is convenient to discuss the ANS and the endocrine/paracrine systems separately, it is important to understand that they do not function independently of one another. Rather, the regulatory systems interact to control secretion, absorption, and motility. Specific examples of such regulation are given in subsequent chapters (see Figures 8-10 and 9-7) for examples. A general scheme of the interaction is depicted in Figure 2-3. The target cells, be they secretory, absorptive, or smooth muscle cells, have a certain resting output that is modulated by both neurally released chemicals and humorally delivered chemicals. These chemicals are released from nerve endings and glandular cells in response to various stimuli that act on specific receptors. The sources of these stimuli can be either in the environment or within the body. For example, seeing or smelling appetizing food alters many aspects of GI function, as does the presence of many foodstuffs and products of digestion within the lumen of the stomach and intestine. In many cases, the stimuli result from the secretory and motor functions of the target cells themselves. Whatever their source, these stimuli initiate inputs that are integrated in the neural and endocrine systems in such a way as to produce outputs that appropriately regulate the functions of the target cells.

E   Endocrine/paracrine

N   Neurocrine

S   Stimulus

— — —   Endocrine pathway

················   Paracrine pathway

FIGURE 2-3 ■ Pathways by which integration of the regulatory systems can occur. Note that most target cells or tissues possess intrinsic activities that are modulated by specific chemicals acting on specific receptors. These chemicals come from nerve endings and endocrine cells. Note also that these same chemicals, as well as the products of the target cells, can alter the activities of the nerves and endocrine cells themselves.

ANATOMY OF THE SMOOTH MUSCLE CELL

The contractile tissue of the GI tract is made up of **smooth muscle cells,** except in the pharynx, orad third of the esophagus, and external anal sphincter. The smooth muscle cells found in each region of the GI tract exhibit functional and structural differences. These special features are considered in subsequent chapters. However, certain basic properties are common to all smooth muscle cells. The cells are small when compared with skeletal muscle cells, being some 4 to 10 micrometers (μm) wide and 50 to 200 μm long. A distinguishing feature of these cells is that the contractile elements are not arranged in orderly sarcomeres as

in skeletal muscle (Figure 2-4). Thus the cells have no striations. Many of the contractile proteins found in striated muscle also exist in smooth muscle, although they differ in isoform and in relative amounts. Actin, along with tropomyosin, is the main constituent of thin filaments, whereas myosin is the main constituent of thick filaments. Compared with skeletal muscle, smooth muscle contains less myosin, much more actin, and little if any troponin. The apparent ratio of thin to thick filaments in smooth muscles is 12:1 to 18:1, rather than 2:1 as in skeletal muscle. In addition to the thick and thin filaments, smooth muscle cells contain a third network of filaments that form an internal "skeleton." These intermediate filaments, along with their associated dense bodies, may serve as anchor points for the

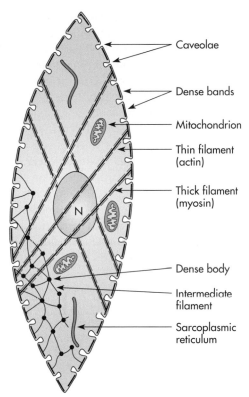

FIGURE 2-4 ■ Intracellular structural specializations of a smooth muscle cell. *(Adapted from Schiller LR: Motor function of the stomach. In Sleisenger MH, Fordtran JS [eds]: Gastrointestinal Disease. Philadelphia, WB Saunders, 1983.)*

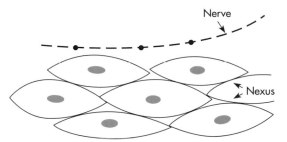

FIGURE 2-5 ■ Anatomic features of "unitary" smooth muscle. Neurotransmitter is released from varicosities along the nerve trunk. Other chemicals arrive via endocrine and paracrine routes. The influence of these substances on one muscle cell is then transmitted to other cells via nexuses.

contractile filaments and may modulate contractile activity.

Smooth muscle cells of the GI tract are grouped into branching bundles, or **fasciae,** that are surrounded by connective tissue sheets. These fasciae, organized into muscular coats, can serve as the effector units because smooth muscle cells of the gut are mostly of the "unitary" type (Figure 2-5). Individual cells are functionally coupled to one another so that the contractions of a bundle of muscle are synchronous. In most tissues, this coupling is due to actual fusion of apposing membranes in the form of gap junctions or nexuses. These junctions serve as areas of low resistance for the spread of excitation from one cell to another. Not every smooth muscle cell is innervated. Nerve axons enter the muscle bundles and release neurotransmitters from swellings along their length.

These swellings usually are some distance from the muscle cells so that no discrete neuromuscular junctions exist. Thus the neurotransmitters probably act on only a few of the muscle cells or on interstitial cells of Cajal, which in turn form junctions with muscle cells. The influence of the transmitters must then be communicated from one smooth muscle cell to the next.

SMOOTH MUSCLE CONTRACTION

There is a remarkable heterogeneity in the time course of contractions among smooth muscles in the GI tract. Some muscles, such as those found in the body of the esophagus, small bowel, and gastric antrum, contract and relax in a matter of seconds (**phasic contractions**). Other smooth muscles, such as those found in the lower esophageal sphincter, orad stomach, and ileocecal and internal anal sphincters, show sustained contractions that last from minutes to hours. These muscles exhibit what are called **tonic contractions**. As discussed in subsequent chapters, the type of contraction, whether phasic or tonic, is governed by the smooth muscle cells themselves or by interstitial cells of Cajal in association with smooth muscle cells. It does not depend on neural or hormonal input. Neurocrines, endocrines, and paracrines are important because they modulate the basic contractile activity, so that the amplitude of the contractions of phasic muscles varies and the tone of the tonic muscles increases or decreases.

As in striated muscle, contractile activity of smooth muscle, especially those muscles that contract phasically, is modulated by fluctuating levels of free intracellular **calcium**. At low levels (less than 10^{-7} molar [M]) of calcium, interaction of the contractile proteins does not occur. At higher levels of calcium, proteins interact and contractions occur. The prevailing theory to explain how calcium brings about contraction is that the calcium, combined with the calcium-binding protein calmodulin, activates a protein kinase that brings about the specific phosphorylation of one of the components of myosin (Figure 2-6). Myosin in its phosphorylated form then interacts with actin to cause contraction, which is fueled by the splitting of **adenosine triphosphate** (ATP). When the intracellular levels of calcium fall, the myosin is dephosphorylated by a specific phosphatase. This brings about a cessation of the interaction between the contractile proteins, and muscle relaxation occurs. In smooth muscles that contract tonically, the exact mechanism for the maintenance of tone is not known. What is known is that tone can be maintained at low levels of phosphorylation of myosin and of ATP utilization. Also, it is becoming apparent that smooth muscle contraction is regulated not only by levels of calcium but also by processes that regulate the activity of the phosphatase(s) that dephosphorylate myosin, thereby altering the calcium sensitivity of the contractile process.

The exact source of the calcium that participates in the contractile process is not certain and appears to vary from one muscle to another. In many muscles (e.g., muscle from the body of the esophagus), calcium enters the cells from the extracellular fluid or from pools of calcium that are tightly bound to the smooth muscle cell membranes or contained in caveolae (see Figure 2-4). Influx of calcium from these sites is regulated by permeability changes of the membrane that also cause characteristic electrical activities (see the following paragraph). In other muscles (e.g., muscle from the lower esophageal sphincter), calcium is sequestered in intracellular structures called the sarcoplasmic reticulum (see Figure 2-4) and is released in response to electrical events of the plasma membrane or to agonist-induced increases in inositol triphosphate, or to both. In addition to these sources for calcium, mechanisms also exist for the expulsion of calcium from the cells and for reuptake into the sarcoplasmic reticulum.

Increases in free intracellular calcium most often are related to electrical activities of the smooth muscle cell membranes. In phasically active muscle, calcium enters the cell by way of voltage-dependent calcium channels. When these are activated, rapid transients in membrane potential occur; these are called **action** or **spike potentials** (see Figure 5-6). In many physically active muscles, these spike potentials do not arise from a stable resting membrane potential. Rather, they are superimposed on relatively slow (3 to 12 cycles/minute) but regular oscillations in membrane potential.

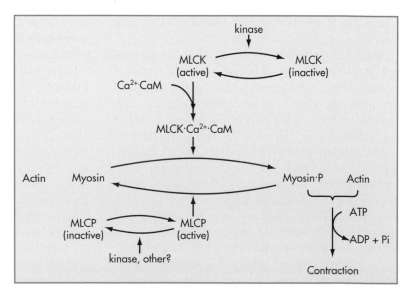

FIGURE 2-6 ■ Biochemical events in smooth muscle contraction. An increase in the levels of Ca^{2+} activates the enzyme myosin light chain kinase (MLCK), which phosphorylates myosin. Phosphorylated myosin (Myosin·P) interacts with actin to cause muscle contraction and ATP consumption. When Ca^{2+} levels fall, the kinase becomes inactive and the activity of myosin light chain phosphatase (MLCP) dominates. Myosin·P is dephosphorylated and the muscle relaxes. The activities of both MLCK and MLCP can be modulated by kinases and/or second messengers to influence calcium sensitivity of the contractile process.

These potential changes, called **slow waves,** do not in themselves cause significant contractions. They set the timing, however, for when spike potentials can occur, because spikes are seen only during the peak of depolarization of the slow wave.

The genesis of slow waves appears to lie in complex interactions among smooth muscle cells and specialized cells called **interstitial cells of Cajal** (ICCs) (Figure 2-7). In all regions of the GI tract from which slow waves are recorded, ICCs are present and are connected to one another to form a three-dimensional network within and/or between the smooth muscle layers. These cells not only communicate with one another but also form gap junctions with smooth muscle cells. Some ICCs

FIGURE 2-7 ■ **Top,** Interactions among interstitial cells of Cajal (ICCs), smooth muscle cells, and nerves. Pacemaker current leading to slow waves appears to originate in the ICC network. Slow waves actively propagate within the ICC network and are passively conducted into the smooth muscle. Other ICCs appear to be interposed between nerve endings and smooth muscle cells; they may be involved in neuromodulation. **Bottom,** Recordings of electrical activity from the small intestine of a normal mouse (A) and a mouse deficient in ICCs (B). Note the absence of slow waves in B. *(Modified from Horowitz B, Ward SM, Sanders KM: Cellular and molecular basis for electrical rhythmicity in gastrointestinal muscles. Annu Rev Physiol 61:19-43, 1999.)*

appear to be interposed between enteric nerve endings and smooth muscle cells and may be involved in neural modulation of smooth muscle activity rather than in slow wave generation. Isolated ICCs exhibit membrane properties that could provide the pacemaker activity responsible for the generation of slow waves. This activity spreads into and affects the smooth muscle cells. Both slow waves and spike potentials are recorded from smooth muscle cells that are coupled to ICCs, but slow waves are absent from intestinal smooth muscle devoid of ICCs (see Figure 2-7).

Slow waves are extremely regular and only minimally influenced by neural or hormonal activities, although they are influenced by body temperature and metabolic activity. The higher the activity, the higher the frequency of slow waves. On the other hand, the occurrence of spike potentials depends heavily on neural and hormonal activities.

An excitatory endocrine, paracrine, or neurocrine will act on a receptor on the smooth muscle cell membrane to induce spike potentials in those cells and in adjacent cells that are coupled to one another. The spike potentials lead to an increase in intercellular free Ca^{++} levels. The Ca^{++} then acts via myosin light chain kinase to induce **contraction**. On the other hand, an inhibitory mediator will act with its receptor on that same membrane. In this case, however, the response will be an inhibition of spike potentials and/or a hyperpolarization of the cell membrane. This results in a decrease in intracellular free Ca^{++} and subsequent **relaxation**. In addition, evidence exists to indicate that activation of cell receptors also can modulate contractile activity through mechanisms not involving the calcium-myosin phosphorylation pathway. Whatever the mechanism, it is the interplay of these excitatory and inhibitory mediators on the basal activity of the muscle that determines the motility functions of the various organs of the gut.

SUMMARY

1. The regulation of GI function results from an interplay of neural and hormonal influences on effector cells that have intrinsic activities.
2. The GI tract is innervated by the ANS, which is composed of nerves that are extrinsic and nerves that are intrinsic to the tract.
3. Extrinsic nerves are distributed to the GI tract through both parasympathetic and sympathetic pathways.
4. Intrinsic nerves are grouped into several nerve plexuses, with the myenteric and submucosal plexuses being the most prominent. Nerves in the plexuses receive input from receptors within the GI tract and from extrinsic nerves. This input can be integrated within the intrinsic nerves such that coordinated activities can be effected.
5. ACh is one of the major excitatory neurotransmitters, and NO and VIP are two of the major inhibitory neurotransmitters at effector cells. Serotonin and somatostatin are two important neurotransmitters of intrinsic interneurons.
6. Striated muscle comprises the musculature of the pharynx, the oral half of the esophagus, and the external anal sphincter. Smooth muscle makes up the musculature of the rest of the GI tract.
7. Adjacent smooth muscle cells are electrically coupled to one another and contract synchronously when stimulated. Some smooth muscles contract tonically, whereas others contract phasically.
8. In phasically active muscle, stimulation induces a rise in intracellular calcium, which in turn induces phosphorylation of the 20,000-dalton light chain of myosin. ATP is split and the muscle contracts as the phosphorylated myosin (myosin-P) interacts with actin. Calcium levels fall, myosin is dephosphorylated, and relaxation occurs. In tonically active muscles, contraction can be maintained at low levels of phosphorylation and ATP utilization.
9. Periodic membrane depolarizations and repolarizations, called slow waves, are major determinants of the phasic nature of contraction. Slow-wave activity is due to ionic currents initiated through the interactions of the ICCs with smooth muscle cells.

KEY WORDS AND CONCEPTS

- Autonomic nervous system
- Extrinsic nervous system
- Parasympathetic innervation
- Sympathetic innervation
- Intrinsic/enteric nervous system
- Myenteric/submucosal plexuses
- Neurocrines
- Acetylcholine
- Norepinephrine
- Serotonin
- Vasoactive intestinal peptide
- Nitric oxide
- Somatostatin
- Substance P
- Smooth muscle cells
- Fasciae
- Phasic contractions
- Tonic contractions
- Calcium
- Adenosine triphosphate
- Action/spike potentials
- Slow waves
- Interstitial cells of Cajal
- Contraction
- Relaxation

REFERENCES

Furness JB, Bornstein JC, Kunze WAA, et al: The enteric nervous system and its extrinsic connections. In Yamada T, Alpers DH, Laine L, et al (eds): Textbook of Gastroenterology, vol 1, 3rd cd. Philadelphia, Lippincott Williams & Wilkins, 1999.

Murphy RA: Muscle in the walls of hollow organs. In Berne RM, Levy MN (eds): Principles of Physiology, 3rd ed. St. Louis, Mosby, 2000.

Pfitzer G: Signal transduction in smooth muscle. Invited review: regulation of myosin phosphorylation in smooth muscle. J Appl Physiol 91:497-503, 2001.

Roman C, Gonella J: Extrinsic control of digestive tract motility. In Johnson LR (ed): Physiology of the Gastrointestinal Tract, vol 1, 2nd ed. New York, Raven Press, 1987.

Sanders KM, Koh SD, Ward SM: Organization and electrophysiology of interstitial cells of Cajal and smooth muscle cells in the gastrointestinal tract. In Johnson LR (ed): Physiology of the Gastrointestinal Tract, 4th ed. San Diego, Elsevier, 2006.

Wood JD: Integrative functions of the enteric nervous system. In Johnson LR (ed): Physiology of the Gastrointestinal Tract, 4th ed. San Diego, Elsevier, 2006.

3

SWALLOWING

NORMAN W. WEISBRODT

The movement of food through the gastrointestinal (GI) tract begins with the food's **oral ingestion**. Once food has been savored, mixed with saliva, and reduced in particle size through the process of chewing, it is propelled to the stomach through the process of swallowing. Swallowing is almost purely a motility function. Little digestion and absorption take place, in part because the transport of material into the stomach takes only seconds.

The process of swallowing involves the integrated contractile activities of the oral cavity, pharynx, esophagus, and orad portion of the stomach. It is initiated by propulsion of material into the oropharynx primarily by movements of the **tongue**. The portion to be swallowed is separated from other material in the mouth so it lies in a chamber created by placing the tip of the tongue against the hard palate (Figure 3-1A). It is propelled by elevation and retraction of the tongue against the palate. As the material passes from the **oral cavity** into the **oropharynx,** the **nasopharynx** is closed by movement of the soft palate and contraction of the superior constrictor muscles of the pharynx (Figure 3-1B). Simultaneously, respiration is inhibited and contraction of the laryngeal muscles closes the **glottis** and raises the **larynx**. The bolus is propelled through the pharynx by a **peristaltic contraction** that begins in the superior constrictor and progresses through the middle and inferior constrictor muscles of the **pharynx** (Figure 3-1C). These contractions, along with relaxation of the **upper esophageal sphincter** (UES), propel the bolus into the esophagus (Figure 3-1D).

The oral and pharyngeal phases of swallowing are rapid, taking less than 1 second. Swallowing can be initiated voluntarily. Once initiated, however, it proceeds as a coordinated involuntary reflex. Coordination is central in origin, and an area within the reticular formation of the brainstem has been identified as the **swallowing center**. Afferent impulses from the pharynx are directed toward this center, which serves to coordinate the activity of other areas of the brain such as the nuclei of the trigeminal, facial, and hypoglossal nerves, as well as the nucleus ambiguus (Figure 3-2). Efferent impulses from the center are distributed to the pharynx via nerves from the nucleus ambiguus. The impulses appear to be sequential, so the pharyngeal musculature is activated in a proximal-to-distal manner. This sequencing accounts for the peristaltic nature of the pharyngeal contractions. The center also appears to interact with other areas of the brain involved with respiration and speech. Injury to the swallowing center produces abnormalities in the pharyngeal component of swallowing.

ESOPHAGEAL PERISTALSIS

The **esophagus** propels material from the pharynx to the stomach. This propulsion is accomplished by coordinated contractions of the muscular layers of the body of the esophagus. Because a large segment of the esophagus is located in the thorax, where the pressure is lower than in the pharynx and stomach, the esophagus also must withstand the entry of air and gastric contents.

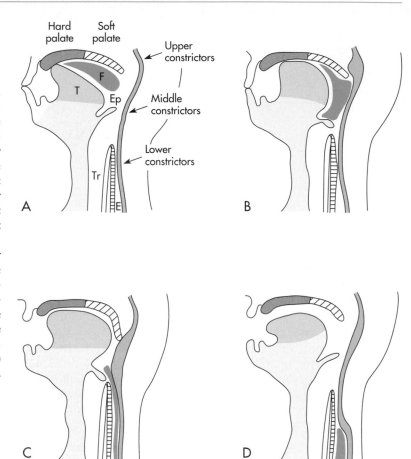

FIGURE 3-1 ■ Oral and pharyngeal events during swallowing. **A,** The food bolus (F) to be swallowed is propelled into the pharynx by placement of the tongue (T) on the roof of the hard palate. **B,** Further propulsion is caused by movement of the more distal regions of the tongue against the palate. Contraction of the upper constrictors of the pharynx and movement of the soft palate separate the oropharynx from the nasopharynx. **C,** Propulsion through the upper esophageal sphincter is accomplished by contraction of the middle and lower constrictors of the pharynx and by relaxation of the cricopharyngeal muscle. Upward movement of the glottis and downward movement of the epiglottis (Ep) seal off the trachea (Tr). **D,** The bolus is now in the esophagus (E) and is propelled into the stomach by a peristaltic contraction.

The barrier functions of the esophagus are accomplished by the presence of sphincters at each end of the organ.

Anatomically the esophageal muscle is arranged in two layers: an inner layer with the muscle fibers organized in a circular axis and an outer layer with the fibers organized in a longitudinal axis. The UES consists of a thickening of the circular muscle and can be identified anatomically as the cricopharyngeal muscle. This muscle, like the musculature of the proximal third of the esophageal body, is striated. The distal third of the esophagus is composed of smooth muscle; although the terminal 1 to 2 centimeters (cm) of the musculature acts as a **lower esophageal sphincter** (LES), no separate sphincter muscle can be identified anatomically. The middle third of the body of the esophagus is composed of a mixture of muscle types with a descending transition from striated to smooth fibers.

The events that occur in the esophagus between and during swallowing are often monitored by placing pressure-sensing devices at various levels in the esophageal lumen. Such devices indicate that between swallows, both the UES and the LES are closed and the body of the esophagus is flaccid (Figure 3-3A). In the region of the UES, pressure is as much as 60 millimeters of mercury (mm Hg) higher than that in the pharynx or body of the esophagus. A zone of elevated pressure also is found at the LES. The length of this zone may range from several millimeters to a few centimeters, and the pressure may be 20 to 40 mm Hg higher than on either side. Pressures in the body of the esophagus are similar to those within the body cavity in which

FIGURE 3-2 ■ Control of pharyngeal and esophageal peristalsis. Sensory input from the pharynx activates an area in the medulla (the swallowing center). This center serves to coordinate activation of the vagal nuclei with other centers such as the respiratory centers. Muscles of the pharynx and striated areas of the esophagus are activated by the center via the nucleus ambiguus. Areas of the smooth muscle are activated via the dorsal motor nucleus. Peristalsis is due to sequential activation of the muscles of the pharynx and esophagus by sequential neural impulses from the center. The *area enclosed within the circle* is shown in more detail in Figure 3-4.

the esophagus lies. In the thorax the pressures are subatmospheric and vary with respiration, dropping with inspiration and rising with expiration. These fluctuations in pressure with respiration reverse below the diaphragm, and intraluminal esophageal pressure reflects intra-abdominal pressure, which is slightly above atmospheric pressure.

During a swallow the sphincters and the body of the esophagus act in a coordinated manner (Figure 3-3B). Shortly before the distal pharyngeal muscles contract, the UES opens. Once the bolus passes, the sphincter closes and assumes its resting tone. The body of the esophagus undergoes a peristaltic contraction.

This contraction begins just below the UES and occurs sequentially at progressively more distal segments to give the appearance of a contractile wave moving toward the stomach. After the contractile sequence passes, the esophageal muscle becomes flaccid again. Shortly before the peristaltic contraction reaches the LES, the sphincter relaxes. After passage of the bolus the sphincter contracts back to its resting level. Compared with the rapid events in the pharynx, esophageal peristalsis is slow. The peristaltic contraction moves down the esophagus at velocities ranging from 2 to 6 cm/second, and it may take the bolus 10 seconds to reach the lower end of the esophagus.

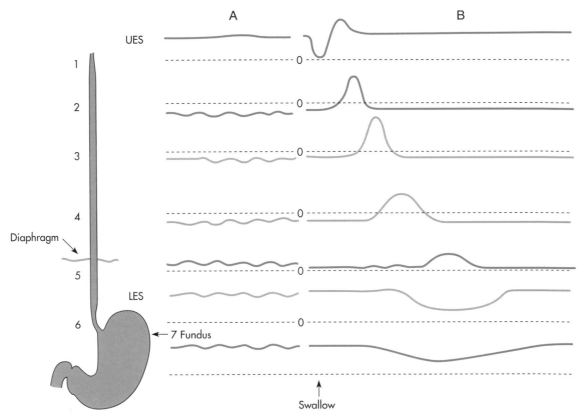

FIGURE 3-3 ■ Manometric recordings from the esophagus and the orad portion of the stomach. Intraluminal pressures from the upper esophageal sphincter, four areas of the esophagus, the lower esophageal sphincter, and the gastric fundus are shown. **A,** Between swallows, both the upper and the lower sphincters are closed, as indicated by the greater than atmospheric pressures recorded there. Pressures in the body of the esophagus reflect intrathoracic or intra-abdominal pressures. Pressures in the fundus reflect intra-abdominal pressure plus tonic contractions of the fundus. **B,** On swallowing, the upper sphincter relaxes before passage of the bolus. After bolus passage it contracts, followed by a peristaltic contraction in the body of the esophagus. To allow passage of the bolus into the stomach, the lower sphincter and the orad stomach relax before the peristaltic contraction reaches them.

When esophageal peristalsis is preceded by a pharyngeal phase, it is called **primary peristalsis.** Esophageal contractions, however, can occur in the absence of both oral and pharyngeal phases. This is called **secondary peristalsis** and is elicited when the esophagus is distended. Secondary peristalsis occurs if the primary contraction fails to empty the esophagus or when gastric contents reflux into the esophagus. Initiation of secondary peristaltic contractions is involuntary and normally is not sensed.

The effect of esophageal peristalsis on bolus transport depends upon the physical properties of the bolus.

If a person in an upright position swallows a liquid bolus, it actually reaches the stomach several seconds before the peristaltic contraction. Thus, although both sphincters must relax to allow transport of all materials, esophageal peristalsis is not always necessary. For most swallowed material, peristaltic contractions are essential for progression to the stomach, and repetitive secondary contractions are often required to sweep the bolus completely into the stomach.

Control of esophageal peristalsis is complex and not fully understood. Closure of the UES is maintained by the normal elasticity of the sphincteric structures and active contraction of the cricopharyngeal muscle. Relaxation of the UES is coordinated with contraction of the pharyngeal musculature. As the larynx rises during the pharyngeal component of swallowing, the cricopharyngeal area is displaced. This displacement, along with relaxation of the cricopharyngeal muscle, allows the sphincter to open. Relaxation of the cricopharyngeal muscle is brought about by a suppression of nerve impulses from the swallowing center via the activity of the nucleus ambiguus.

Contractions of the body of the esophagus are coordinated by both central and peripheral mechanisms. This region of the esophagus is innervated primarily by the vagus nerves. These nerves are partly of the somatic motor type, arising from the nucleus ambiguus, and partly of the visceral motor type, arising from the dorsal motor nucleus. The somatic motor nerves synapse directly with striated muscle fibers of the esophagus (Figure 3-4). The visceral motor nerves do not synapse directly with the smooth muscle cells but rather with nerve cell bodies that lie between the longitudinal and circular muscle layers. These local nerves, in turn, innervate the smooth muscle cells as well as communicate with one another along the length of the esophagus.

Central control of swallowing originates within the swallowing center, which sends a series of sequential impulses to progressively more distal segments of the esophagus. This sequential activation results in a peristaltic contraction. The central nervous system does not totally control peristalsis, however. In smooth muscle areas of the esophagus, peristalsis can occur after bilateral cervical **vagotomy** (cutting of the vagus nerve). Furthermore, peristalsis can be induced in excised esophagi that have been placed in an organ bath. In these instances, peristalsis must be coordinated by the intrinsic nerve plexuses or the smooth muscle cells themselves.

The presence of secondary peristalsis indicates the importance of afferent input to the central and peripheral mechanisms controlling swallowing. Afferent input provided by distention of the esophagus not only initiates secondary peristalsis, it also affects the intensity of contractions. Variation in the size of the bolus being swallowed leads to a variation in the amplitude of esophageal contraction. Indeed, afferent stimulation appears so important that a peristaltic sequence may not occur unless a bolus is swallowed and elicits afferent

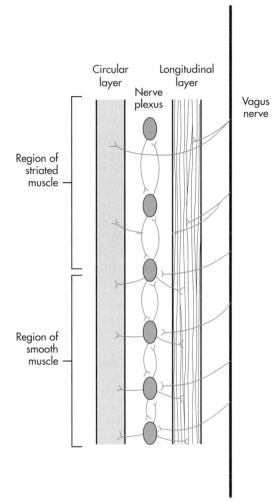

FIGURE 3-4 ■ Efferent innervation of the body of the esophagus. Special visceral somatic fibers directly innervate the striated muscle fibers of the circular and longitudinal muscle layers. Preganglionic fibers from the vagus innervate the ganglion cells of the intrinsic plexus. Fibers from the ganglion cells then innervate the smooth muscle cells of both layers. In addition, the ganglion cells have neural connections with one another.

stimulation. On the other hand, intense afferent stimulation, such as that provided by inflation of a balloon in the body of the esophagus, can inhibit the progression of peristaltic contractions past the balloon.

Contraction of the LES is regulated by the intrinsic properties of the smooth muscle fibers, as well as by neural and humoral influences. Smooth muscle from this area of the esophagus responds to passive stretching by contracting to oppose the stretch. This response does not depend on nervous activity. Thus the basic tone of the LES may be totally myogenic. Nevertheless, this tone is under a number of neural and humoral influences. For example, resting tone is increased by cholinergic agonists and by the GI hormone gastrin. Sphincteric tone is decreased by agents such as isoproterenol and prostaglandin E_1.

Transient relaxation of the LES during swallowing is mediated through enteric nerves. The enteric inhibitory nerves can be activated by stimulation of the vagus nerve and by distention of the body of the esophagus, thus activating aborad enteric nerves. The neurochemical basis for this response is not known, although roles for both vasoactive intestinal peptide (VIP) and nitric oxide (NO) have been proposed.

RECEPTIVE RELAXATION OF THE STOMACH

Swallowing also involves the stomach. In terms of motility functions, the stomach can be divided into two major areas: the **orad portion,** which consists of the fundus and a portion of the body, and the **caudad portion,** which consists of the distal body and the antrum (Figure 3-5). These two regions have markedly different patterns of motility that are responsible, in part, for two major functions: accommodation of ingested material during swallowing, and regulation of gastric emptying. Accommodation is attributable primarily to activities of the oral region, whereas both regions are involved in the regulation of gastric emptying (see Chapter 4).

During a swallow, the orad region of the stomach relaxes at about the same time as the LES. Intraluminal pressures in both regions fall before arrival of the swallowed bolus because of active relaxation of the smooth muscle in both regions (see Figure 3-3B). After passage of the bolus, the pressure in the stomach returns to approximately what it was before the swallow. This process has been termed **receptive relaxation**. Because relaxation happens with each swallow, large volumes can be accommodated with a minimal rise in intragastric pressure. For example, the human stomach can accept 1600 cubic centimeters (cc) of air with a rise in pressure of no more than 10 mm Hg.

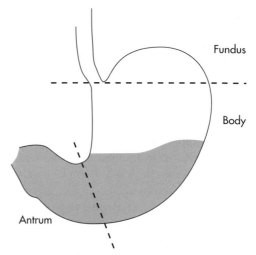

FIGURE 3-5 ■ Divisions of the stomach. For discussions of secretion, the stomach usually is divided into the fundus, body, and antrum. For discussions of motility, it can be divided into an orad area and a caudad area. *Shading* denotes the approximate extent of the caudad area.

Receptive relaxation is mediated by a nervous reflex that has its afferent and efferent pathways in the vagus nerve. If this nerve is transected, receptive relaxation is impaired and the stomach becomes less distendible. The neurotransmitters that mediate receptive relaxation are unknown, but NO may again be involved.

CLINICAL APPLICATIONS

Contractions of pharyngeal muscle are controlled solely by extrinsic nerves. Therefore certain neurologic diseases (such as cerebrovascular accident) can have an adverse effect on this phase of swallowing. Aspiration often occurs because contractions in the pharynx and UES are no longer coordinated. A similar clinical picture can be seen in diseases that affect striated muscle or the myoneural junction.

Diseases affecting the smooth muscle portion of the esophagus predictably cause abnormalities in peristalsis and in the tone of the LES. In **achalasia,** for example, the LES often fails to relax completely with swallowing. This may be coupled with a loss of peristalsis in the esophageal body, a complete absence of contractions, or the appearance of simultaneous rather than sequential contractions, resulting in impaired transit.

Patients with this disorder have considerable difficulty swallowing, often aspirate retained esophageal content, and may become severely malnourished. This disorder has been attributed to abnormalities in the enteric nerves. In another disorder, **diffuse esophageal spasm,** simultaneous contractions of a long duration and high amplitude can occur. Affected persons have difficulty swallowing and may complain of chest pain. Although not always symptomatic, abnormalities in the esophageal component of swallowing can occur as part of a variety of systemic diseases. Examples are diabetes mellitus, chronic alcoholism, and scleroderma.

Motor dysfunction also can play an important contributory role in the pathogenesis of other esophageal diseases. One common example is **acid injury to the esophageal mucosa,** which results from reflux of gastric contents. Often underlying this problem are abnormally low resting pressure, inappropriate transient relaxations of the LES, and poor or ineffective secondary peristalsis in the esophageal body. The causes of these motor abnormalities are unknown.

CLINICAL TESTS

Swallowing is assessed clinically by x-ray examination with barium and by esophageal manometry. In the x-ray study the patient swallows a bolus of liquid barium sulfate. This material is radiopaque and thus can be observed fluoroscopically and recorded on the x-ray film as it traverses the esophagus, thereby providing a qualitative description of motor events in both the pharynx and the esophagus.

If a more detailed description of events is required or there is a suspicion of motor disorders such as those just described, esophageal manometry is often useful. Catheters are passed through the nose or mouth so that their tips lie in various regions of the esophagus. Pressures detected by the catheters then are recorded between and during swallowing small sips of water, thus providing a quantitative description of events occurring in the sphincters and body of the esophagus.

A useful test for episodes of acid reflux is 24-hour monitoring of intraesophageal pH. A small pH probe is inserted nasally and positioned 5 cm above the LES. A small battery-powered computer is used for continuous recordings of pH.

SUMMARY

1. Swallowing is initiated voluntarily, but once initiated, it proceeds as an involuntary reflex.
2. Swallowing is accomplished by peristaltic contraction of pharyngeal muscles, during which time the UES relaxes. This is followed by peristaltic contraction of the esophageal musculature, during which time the LES and the orad region of the stomach relax.
3. Peristaltic contraction of the pharyngeal muscles, relaxation of the UES, and peristaltic contraction of the striated muscle of the upper esophagus are regulated by pathways within the central nervous system. Peristaltic contraction of the smooth muscle of the lower esophagus and relaxation of the LES are regulated by pathways within the central nervous system and by pathways within the intrinsic nerves.
4. Contraction of the pharynx and esophagus can be initiated by swallowing (primary peristalsis). Contraction of the esophagus can be initiated by stimulation of receptors within the esophagus (secondary peristalsis).
5. Tonic contraction of the LES between swallows is due to an interplay of excitatory and inhibitory neural and hormonal influences acting on an intrinsic myogenic contraction. During a swallow, intrinsic nerves release a transmitter (perhaps NO or VIP) to cause muscle relaxation.
6. Contraction of the orad stomach is due to an interplay of excitatory and inhibitory neural and

hormonal influences acting on an intrinsic myogenic contraction. During a swallow, the orad stomach relaxes (receptive relaxation) due to activation of inhibitory nerves in the vagus.

KEY WORDS AND CONCEPTS

- Oral ingestion
- Tongue
- Oral cavity
- Oropharynx
- Nasopharynx
- Glottis
- Larynx
- Peristaltic contraction
- Pharynx
- Upper esophageal sphincter
- Swallowing center
- Esophagus
- Lower esophageal sphincter
- Primary peristalsis

- Secondary peristalsis
- Vagotomy
- Orad region
- Caudad region
- Receptive relaxation
- Achalasia
- Diffuse esophageal spasm
- Acid injury to the esophageal mucosa

REFERENCES

Biancani P, Harnett KM, Behar J: Esophageal motor function. In Yamada T, Alpers DH, Laine L, et al (eds): Textbook of Gastroenterology, vol 1, 3rd ed. Philadelphia, Lippincott Williams & Wilkins, 1999.

Clouse RE, Diamant NE: Motor functions of the esophagus. In Johnson LR (ed): Physiology of the Gastrointestinal Tract, vol 1, 4th ed. San Diego, Elsevier, 2006.

Roman C, Gonella J: Extrinsic control of digestive tract motility. In Johnson LR (ed): Physiology of the Gastrointestinal Tract, vol 1, 2nd ed. New York, Raven Press, 1987.

Shaker R: Pharyngeal motor function. In Johnson LR (ed): Physiology of the Gastrointestinal Tract, vol 1, 4th ed. San Diego, Elsevier, 2006.

4

GASTRIC EMPTYING

NORMAN W. WEISBRODT

Motility of the stomach and upper small intestine is organized to accomplish the orderly emptying of contents into the duodenum in the face of variable quantity and composition of ingested material. Accommodation and temporary storage of ingested material result from receptive relaxation of the orad stomach (see Chapter 3). Emptying, which also requires mixing ingested material with gastric juice and reducing the particle size of any solids that have been swallowed, results from integrated contractions of the orad stomach, caudad stomach, pylorus, and duodenum.

ANATOMIC CONSIDERATIONS

Gastric contractions result from activity of smooth muscle cells that are arranged in three layers: an outer longitudinal layer, a middle circular layer, and an inner oblique layer. The **longitudinal layer** is absent on the anterior and posterior surfaces of the stomach. The **circular layer** is the most prominent and is present in all areas of the stomach except the paraesophageal region. The **oblique layer** is the least complete, being formed from two bands of muscle lying on the anterior and posterior surfaces. These two bands meet at the gastroesophageal sphincter and fan out to fuse with the circular muscle layer in the caudad part of the stomach. Both the circular and the longitudinal muscle layers increase in thickness toward the duodenum.

The stomach is richly innervated with both intrinsic and extrinsic nerves. The intrinsic nerves lie in various plexuses, the most prominent being the myenteric plexus, which lies in a three-dimensional matrix between the longitudinal and circular muscle layers and throughout the circular muscle layer. The myenteric plexus receives nerve endings from other intrinsic plexuses, as well as from extrinsic nerves. Axons from neurons within the myenteric plexus synapse with the muscle fibers and with glandular cells of the stomach. Extrinsically the stomach is innervated by branches of the vagus nerves and by fibers originating in the celiac plexus of the sympathetic nervous system.

The **pylorus,** or gastroduodenal junction, is characterized by a thickening of the circular muscle layer of the distal antrum. Separating this bundle of muscle from the duodenum is a connective tissue septum; however, some of the longitudinal muscle fibers pass from the antrum to connect with muscle cells of the duodenum. The pylorus is richly innervated with both extrinsic and intrinsic nerves, and nerve endings within the thickened circular muscle layer are abundant. Many of these endings contain neuropeptides, especially enkephalin, and many produce and release nitric oxide (NO).

The anatomy of the proximal duodenum is similar to that of the rest of the intestine (described in Chapter 5). A significant difference is the larger number of intrinsic nerves present in this area compared with the rest of the small bowel. These may be involved in the regulation of gastric emptying (described in a later section).

In addition to the muscle cells and nerves, interstitial cells of Cajal (ICCs) also are prominent in all regions and appear to play a prominent role in regulating motility. Many ICCs form gap junctions with smooth muscle cells, whereas others appear to bridge between nerve endings and smooth muscle cells.

CONTRACTIONS OF THE ORAD REGION OF THE STOMACH

As detailed in the previous chapter, the predominant motor activity of the orad region of the stomach is the accommodation of ingested material. During the remainder of the digestive state, pressures in the orad stomach are essentially equal to intra-abdominal pressure, with superimposed tonic pressure changes. These pressure changes are predominantly of low amplitude and have durations of 1 minute or more. The contractions that produce these pressure changes reduce the size of the stomach as the stomach empties. These tonic contractions result in accommodation of the remaining gastric contents and propulsion of those contents into the caudad stomach. A consequence of this minimal contractile activity is that little mixing of ingested contents occurs in the orad stomach. Contents often remain in relatively undisturbed layers for an hour or more after eating. Little is known about the regulation of contractions in the orad stomach during digestion. Both gastrin and cholecystokinin (CCK) decrease contractions and increase gastric distensibility. However, only the effect of CCK appears to be physiologic.

CONTRACTIONS OF THE CAUDAD REGION OF THE STOMACH

Compared with the orad stomach, the caudad region exhibits marked activity. After eating, phasic contractions of variable intensity occur almost continuously. Contractions normally begin in the midstomach and move toward the gastroduodenal junction (Figure 4-1). Thus the primary contractile event is a **peristaltic contraction.** As contractions approach the gastroduodenal junction, they increase in both force and velocity. At any one locus of the human stomach, the duration of each contraction ranges between 2 and 20 seconds, and the maximum frequency is approximately three contractions per minute. Between contractions, pressures in the caudad region are near intra-abdominal levels.

Contractions of the caudad region of the stomach serve to both mix and propel gastric contents. Once a contraction begins in the midportion of the stomach, gastric contents are propelled toward the gastroduodenal

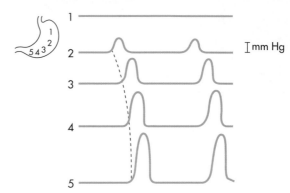

FIGURE 4-1 ■ Intraluminal pressures recorded from five areas of the stomach. A sensor in the orad region records little phasic activity. Sensors in the caudad region detect peristaltic contractions, which begin in the midportion of the stomach and progress toward the gastroduodenal junction. The contractions increase in force and velocity as they near the junction, and they repeat at multiple intervals of 12 to 20 seconds. The presence and force of contractions depend on the digestive state of the individual.

junction (Figure 4-2A). As the contraction approaches the gastroduodenal junction, some contents are evacuated into the duodenum (Figure 4-2B). However, because the peristaltic wave increases in velocity as it approaches the junction, the contraction overtakes the gastric contents. Once this occurs, most of the contents are propelled back into the main body of the stomach (Figure 4-2C), where they remain until the next contraction sequence (Figure 4-2D). This propulsion back into the stomach has been termed **retropulsion.** Retropulsion causes a thorough mixing of the gastric contents and mechanically reduces the size of solid particles. (See videos: http://www.wzw.tum.de/humanbiology/motvid01/movie_11_1mot01.wmv; http://www.wzw.tum.de/humanbiology/motvid01/movie_13_1mot01.wmv)

Contractions of the caudad area of the stomach are controlled by interactions among smooth muscle cells and ICCs, as well as by nervous and humoral elements. Smooth muscle cells in this area have a membrane potential that fluctuates rhythmically with cyclic depolarizations and repolarizations. These fluctuations are called **slow waves** (also referred to as *basic electric rhythm, pacesetter potentials,* and *control activity*). Slow waves have two components: an initial upstroke potential and a secondary plateau potential. In the stomach, slow

FIGURE 4-2 ■ Effects that gastric peristaltic contractions have on intraluminal contents. **A,** The contraction begins in the midregion of the stomach and pushes contents toward the duodenum. **B,** As the contraction increases in force and velocity, some of the contents are passed over and forced back into the body of the stomach. **C,** Contraction force and velocity are great enough to cause rapid and almost complete closure of the distal antrum. Before and during this contraction, a portion of the contents is propelled into the duodenum. However, most of the contents is propelled back into the body of the stomach. **D,** No gross movement of the gastric contents occurs between contractions.

waves can initiate significant contractions; thus some investigators refer to them as *action potentials*. However, slow waves are always present, regardless of the presence or absence of contractions. Their frequency is constant and in humans is approximately 3 cycles/minute (cpm). If slow waves are recorded from multiple sites between the midstomach and the gastroduodenal junction, they have the same frequency at all sites (Figure 4-3). However, slow waves do not occur simultaneously at all points along the stomach. Rather, a phase lag occurs; thus, they seem to pass from an area in the midstomach toward the gastroduodenal junction. This phase lag between slow waves at equidistant points lessens as the gastroduodenal junction is neared. The frequency and velocity of the peristaltic waves are therefore controlled by the frequency and velocity of spread of the slow wave.

Nervous and humoral factors are not necessary for the presence of slow waves, but they do alter slow wave behavior. Vagotomy disorganizes the slow waves so that the phase lag varies in both duration and direction. The hormone gastrin increases the frequency of gastric slow waves while having little effect on their apparent propagation through the musculature.

Simultaneous recordings of both electrical and mechanical activities have shown that slow waves initiate

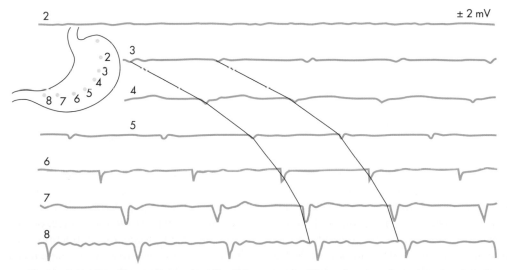

FIGURE 4-3 ■ Electrical activity of smooth muscle cells of the stomach. Electrodes placed on the serosal surface record no changes from the orad region. In the midregion, however, slow waves occur continuously at intervals of 12 to 20 seconds. Slow waves give the appearance of moving through the caudad region at increasing velocities. Compare this with Figure 4-1. mV, microvolts. *(Adapted from Kelly KA, Code CF, Elveback LR: Patterns of canine gastric electrical activity. Am J Physiol 217:461-471, 1969.)*

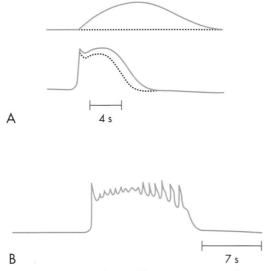

A   4 s

B   7 s

FIGURE 4-4 ■ **A,** Relationship between electrical and mechanical activities of smooth muscle from the caudad region of the stomach. *Bottom tracing* depicts two slow waves (action potentials) superimposed. *Top tracing* depicts mechanical events associated with the potential changes. Note that a contraction is initiated only by the slow wave of larger amplitude and longer duration. **B,** Slow wave potential recorded from distal antrum. Note the oscillations and spike potentials during plateau. s, seconds. *(**A,** Adapted from Szurszewski JH: Mechanism of action of pentagastrin and acetylcholine on the longitudinal muscle of the canine antrum. J Physiol 252:335-361, 1975. **B,** Adapted from El-Sharkaway TY, Morgan KG, Szurszewski JH: Intracellular electrical activity of canine and human gastric smooth muscle. J Physiol 279:291-307, 1978.)*

significant contractions of the musculature only when the plateau potential exceeds a threshold (Figure 4-4). Once the threshold is exceeded, the greater the amplitude of the plateau, the greater will be the force of contraction. The plateau potential may or may not be accompanied by superimposed rapid oscillations called **spike potentials** or **spike bursts.** These oscillations also appear to initiate contractions and are seen more frequently in muscle of the caudad antrum. Threshold values for contraction are not reached by every slow wave. Therefore not every slow wave is accompanied by a contraction. If the threshold is reached, it is only during a specific phase of the slow wave cycle. Thus the phasic and peristaltic nature of

gastric contractions results from the presence of slow waves.

The amplitude of the plateau potential and therefore the number and force of contractions are markedly influenced by nervous and humoral activities. Vagal nerve transection leads to a decrease in contractions, whereas vagal stimulation increases the number and force of contractions. Usually, sympathetic nerve activity depresses contractions. Some hormones, such as gastrin and motilin, increase contractions, whereas others, such as somatostatin, secretin, and gastric inhibitory peptide (GIP), inhibit them. The physiologic significance of these actions is not known.

CONTRACTIONS OF THE GASTRODUODENAL JUNCTION

The question of whether a true sphincter exists between the stomach and duodenum is unsettled. There is a definite difference in the contractile activities of the stomach, on one side, and of the duodenum, on the other. One contracts at a frequency of around 3 cpm, and the other at around 12 cpm. The thickened ring of circular muscle between the two organs appears to behave independently. In humans, some investigators have demonstrated a zone of elevated pressure between the stomach and the duodenum (an indication of sphincteric activity); others, however, have not found such an area. Recent studies show that even if a zone of elevated pressure is not found, the pylorus can contract independently, thus altering the resistance to flow between the stomach and duodenum (Figure 4-5). This can have a large effect on gastric emptying.

CONTRACTIONS OF THE PROXIMAL DUODENUM

Duodenal contractions are mostly phasic. Although their maximum frequency can be around 12 per minute in the digestive state, they seldom occur in a continuous manner. Rather, single, isolated contractions, or small groups of contractions, separated by intervals of no contractions, are the norm. Also, duodenal contractions are not always peristaltic. Most contractions of the small intestine are of the segmenting type (see Chapter 5). Thus, depending on their number and pattern, duodenal contractions either

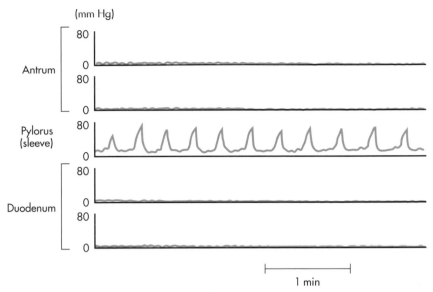

(mm Hg)

Antrum

Pylorus
(sleeve)

Duodenum

1 min

FIGURE 4-5 ■ Intraluminal pressures recorded from two areas of the stomach (antrum), the pylorus, and two areas of the proximal duodenum during the intraduodenal infusion of lipid. Note the regular isolated contractions, and the elevated pressures (0 indicates atmospheric pressure in each tracing) between contractions, in the pylorus. This activity is occurring at a time when no contractions are present in the stomach and duodenum (*min*, minute). *(Adapted from Heddle R, Dent J, Read NW, et al: Antropyloroduodenal motor responses to intraduodenal lipid infusion in healthy volunteers. Am J Physiol 254:G671-G679, 1988.)*

impede or facilitate the emptying of contents from the stomach.

REGULATION OF GASTRIC EMPTYING

Immediately after ingestion of a meal, the stomach may contain over a liter of material, which takes several hours to leave the stomach and empty into the small intestine. Gastric emptying is accomplished by coordinated contractile activity of the stomach, pylorus, and proximal small intestine (Figure 4-6). Emptying appears to be regulated in a manner that allows for optimal intestinal digestion and absorption of foodstuffs (Figure 4-7). Solids empty only after a lag period during which they are reduced in size by retropulsive activity of the caudad stomach. Only particles around 1 mm³ or less in size are readily emptied during the digestive phase of gastric motility. On the other hand, liquids begin to empty almost immediately. The rate of emptying of both solids and liquids depends on their chemical compositions. Materials that are high in lipids or H^+ or that deviate

markedly from isotonicity all empty at a slower rate than that observed for near-isotonic saline solutions.

Regulation of emptying results from the presence of receptors that lie in the upper small bowel. These receptors appear to respond to the physical properties (e.g., osmotic pressure) and chemical composition (e.g., H^+, lipids) of the intestinal contents. As contents empty from the stomach, **intestinal receptors** are activated. Receptor activation in turn results in an inhibition of emptying through pathways that are not completely understood. Many of the substances that inhibit gastric emptying also release one or more **gastrointestinal** (GI) **hormones,** and many of the hormones slow gastric emptying when injected. Thus it is tempting to speculate that foodstuffs inhibit emptying by releasing hormones. However, such a causal relationship has been hard to establish. It is just as likely that these receptors regulate emptying through neural mechanisms.

Regulation of gastric emptying is brought about by alterations in the motility of the stomach, gastroduodenal junction, and duodenum. Decreases in distensibility of the orad stomach, increases in the force of

A   B   C

FIGURE 4-6 ■ Regulation of gastric emptying. **A,** Hypothetical conditions immediately after the rapid ingestion of a meal and before the onset of any contractile activity. This outline is superimposed in **B** and **C** to illustrate changes. **B,** Conditions favoring emptying are increased tone of the orad region of the stomach, forceful peristaltic contractions of the caudad region of the stomach, relaxation of the pylorus, and absence of segmenting contractions of the duodenum. As nutrients emptied from the stomach are further digested and absorbed in the small intestine, they excite receptors located in the intestinal mucosa. Activation of these receptors results in **C. C,** Relaxation of the orad region of the stomach, a decrease in the number and force of contractions of the caudad region of the stomach, contraction of the pylorus, and an increase in segmenting contractions of the duodenum. This results in a slowing of gastric emptying.

peristaltic contractions of the caudad stomach, increases in diameter and inhibition of contractions of the pylorus, and inhibition of segmenting contractions of the proximal duodenum all lead to an increase in the rate of gastric emptying. On activation of the duodenal receptors, one or more of these contractile activities of the stomach and duodenum are reversed to slow emptying (see Figure 4-6). (See videos: http://www.wzw.tum.de/humanbiology/motvid01/

movie_09_1mot01.wmv;http://www.wzw.tum.de/humanbiology/motvid01/movie_45_1mot01.wmv)

The pattern of motility of the gastroduodenal area changes after the nutrient components of the meal have been digested and absorbed. Any large particles of undigested residue that remain in the stomach are emptied by a burst of peristaltic contractions (phase 3) as part of the migrating motor complex (MMC) (Figure 4-8). During this short burst, powerful contractions begin in

FIGURE 4-7 ■ Solid and liquid components of a meal were labeled so that their emptying from the stomach could be followed over time after ingestion of the meal. As indicated by the sharp decrease in the fraction remaining in the stomach, the liquid component began to empty almost immediately; it also emptied more rapidly. On the other hand, there was a lag time before the emptying of the label attached to the solid component, and this label emptied more slowly. This slower emptying was due to the fact that the solid component had to be reduced to small particles before being emptied into the duodenum. *(Adapted from Camilleri M, Malagelada JR, Brown ML, et al: Relation between antral motility and gastric emptying of solids and liquids in humans. Am J Physiol 249: G580-G585, 1985.)*

Proximal stomach

Transitional area

Antrum (orad)

Antrum (mid)

Antrum (caudad)

Duodenum

FIGURE 4-8 ■ Schematic of intraluminal pressures recorded from the stomach and proximal duodenum during an active phase of an MMC. Note that phasic contractions begin in the orad region of the stomach and propagate over the caudad region. As contractions of the caudad region approach the gastroduodenal junction, the pylorus relaxes *(not shown)* and duodenal contractions are momentarily inhibited. This allows contents to be swept into the duodenum. Contents are then propelled toward the colon, as described in Chapter 5. *(Adapted from Malagelada JR, Azpiroz F: Determinants of gastric emptying and transit in the small intestine. In Schultz SG, Wood JD, Rauner BB [eds]: The Gastrointestinal System, vol 1. Bethesda, MD, American Physiological Society, 1989.)*

the previously inactive orad region and sweep the entire length of the stomach. The pylorus dilates and the duodenum relaxes during each sweep so that the resistance to emptying is minimal. Then **duodenal contractions** sweep the contents onward (see Chapter 5). (See video:http://www.wzw.tum.de/humanbiology/motvid02/movie_06_1mot02.wmv) After a burst of activity, the region remains relaxed for an hour or more. Then intermittent contractions begin and lead to another burst. This cycle repeats every 90 minutes or so until ingestion of the next meal. Premature bursts can be initiated by injection of the hormone motilin and by drugs (e.g., erythromycin) thought to act on motilin receptors.

CLINICAL APPLICATIONS

Disorders of gastric motility generally are manifested by a rate of gastric emptying that is either too slow or too fast. This may reflect an abnormality in one or all of the major motor functions of the stomach. When the stomach fails to empty properly, the affected person experiences nausea, loss of appetite, and early satiety, and gastric contents often may be vomited. The most

common cause of impaired emptying is obstruction at the gastric outlet. Examples of disorders that may result in obstruction are gastric cancer and peptic ulcer disease. In the latter, the gastric lumen at the pylorus may actually become occluded from inflammation and scarring associated with the ulcer. Impaired emptying also can be caused by the absence or disorganization of motor events in the caudad stomach. These phenomena occur with a variety of metabolic disorders, such as diabetes mellitus and potassium depletion.

Vagus nerve section (**vagotomy**) invariably leads to a delay in gastric emptying of solids. Consequently, vagotomy (e.g., performed to decrease acid secretion in peptic ulcer disease) is coupled with surgical alterations of the pylorus (**pyloroplasty**) or creation of a new gastric outlet (**gastroenterostomy**) in an attempt to avoid this complication. After such an operation, emptying of liquids generally is accelerated, but even with alteration of the gastric outlet, emptying of solids still may be slowed. A majority of patients undergoing this type of surgery experience no other symptoms. However, some may experience diarrhea, sweating, palpitations, cramps, and a variety of other unpleasant symptoms, all of which result from changes in gastric emptying.

It is speculated that motility abnormalities may underlie or contribute to other diseases of the upper GI tract. For example, gastric emptying is accelerated in patients with a duodenal ulcer; this accelerated emptying may enhance the delivery of gastric acid to the duodenum, perhaps overwhelming the ability of the duodenal mucosa to defend itself against injury. Alternatively, for patients with a gastric ulcer, gastric emptying appears to be slowed. This slowing may create a situation in which the stomach is more susceptible to injury.

CLINICAL TESTS

A qualitative assessment of gastric motility and emptying can be obtained by x-ray and fluoroscopic evaluation of a barium-filled stomach. Aspiration of the stomach at specific intervals after instillation of an isotonic saline solution also gives information regarding gastric emptying. A more quantitative test involves gamma-scintigraphy. For this test, radiolabeled liquid and/or solid food is ingested, and gamma cameras are used to scan the stomach at various times afterward. The fraction of material remaining in the stomach is then plotted as a function of time (see Figure 4-7). In certain laboratories, manometry like that used to assess esophageal motility can be employed. Compliance of the orad stomach can be assessed using a "barostat," a large bag placed in the stomach that monitors changes in volume under set pressures. More recently, magnetic resonance imaging (MRI) and ultrasonography are being employed as noninvasive methods.

SUMMARY

1. Contractile activity of the orad stomach varies with the digestive state. After the orad region has accommodated a meal, it exhibits low-amplitude, long-lasting contractions as the meal empties. After the meal has been digested and absorbed, the orad stomach undergoes periodic bursts of high-amplitude contractions as part of the MMC.

2. Contractions of the caudad stomach are mostly peristaltic, beginning in the midstomach and progressing toward the duodenum. During emptying of a meal, contractions are of variable amplitude and are more or less continuous at a frequency of about 3 cpm. During the interdigestive period, forceful peristaltic contractions are grouped into periodic bursts as part of the MMC.

3. Gastric emptying is highly regulated and involves feedback inhibition from receptors located in the upper small intestine. Receptors are stimulated by osmotic pressure, H^+, and fatty acids. Stimulation results in patterns of motility that slow emptying: decreased tonic contraction of the orad stomach, decreased force and number of contractions of the caudad stomach, increased tone and phasic contractions of the pylorus, and increased segmenting contractions of the upper duodenum.

4. Rhythmic membrane depolarizations and repolarizations called slow waves occur in smooth muscle cells of the caudad stomach. They are omnipresent, occurring at a frequency of about three per minute. Each depolarization appears to be initiated first in the midstomach and then to propagate toward the pylorus. Slow waves appear to set the timing and the peristaltic nature of contractions; however, not every slow wave initiates a contraction. Those that do are of large amplitude and may exhibit superimposed spike potentials.

5. Vagotomy results in a decrease in the number and force of contractions of the caudad stomach and a decrease in gastric emptying of solids. Motilin induces contractions that are part of the gastric phase of the MMC.

KEY WORDS AND CONCEPTS

- Longitudinal layer
- Circular layer

- Oblique layer
- Pylorus
- Peristaltic contraction
- Retropulsion
- Slow waves
- Spike potentials/spike bursts
- Intestinal receptors
- Gastrointestinal hormones
- Duodenal contractions
- Vagotomy
- Pyloroplasty
- Gastroenterostomy

REFERENCES

Ehrlein HJ, Akkermans LMA: Gastric emptying. In Akkermans LMA, Johnson AG, Read NW (eds): Gastric and Gastroduodenal Motility. New York, Praeger, 1984.

Hasler WL: The physiology of gastric motility and gastric emptying. In Yamada T, Alpers DH, Laine L, et al (eds): Textbook of Gastroenterology, vol 1, 3rd ed. Philadelphia, Lippincott Williams & Wilkins, 1999.

Hunt JN, Knox MT: Regulation of gastric emptying. In Code CF (ed): Handbook of Physiology, vol 4. Baltimore, Williams & Wilkins, 1968.

Mayer EA: The physiology of gastric storage and emptying. In Johnson LR (ed): Physiology of the gastrointestinal tract, vol 1, 3rd ed. New York, Raven Press, 1994.

5 MOTILITY OF THE SMALL INTESTINE

NORMAN W. WEISBRODT

Motility of the small intestine is organized to optimize the processes of digestion and absorption of nutrients and the aboral propulsion of undigested material. Thus, contractions perform at least three functions: (1) mixing of ingested foodstuffs with digestive secretions and enzymes, (2) circulation of all intestinal contents to facilitate contact with the intestinal mucosa, and (3) net propulsion of the intestinal contents in an aboral direction.

ANATOMIC CONSIDERATIONS

Contractions of the small intestine are effected by the activities of two layers of smooth muscle cells: an outer layer with the long axis of the cells arranged longitudinally and an inner layer with the long axis of the cells arranged circularly. In general, the circular muscle layer is thicker, and both layers are more abundant in the proximal intestine, decreasing in thickness distally to the level of the ileocecal junction.

The small intestine is richly innervated by elements of the autonomic nervous system. Within the wall of the intestine itself lie neurons, nerve endings, and receptors of the enteric nervous system (see Figure 2-2). These neural elements tend to be concentrated in several plexuses. The most prominent, the **myenteric** or **Auerbach plexus,** lies between the circular and longitudinal layers of smooth muscle cells. Plexal neurons receive input from other neurons within the plexus, from receptors located in the mucosa and muscle walls, and from the central nervous system by way of the parasympathetic and sympathetic nerve trunks. Plexal neurons provide integrated output to smooth muscle cells of both muscle layers, to epithelial cells, and perhaps to endocrine and immune cells. Many neurotransmitters are present in the enteric nervous system, including acetylcholine, norepinephrine, vasoactive intestinal peptide, enkephalin, and other peptides. Furthermore, many nerves express nitric oxide synthase activity.

Interstitial cells of Cajal (ICCs) also are prominent in and adjacent to the enteric nerves and muscular layers of the intestine. At least two major classes of ICCs have been identified: those responsible for generating slow waves and those involved in mediating neural input to the smooth muscle cells.

Extrinsic innervation is supplied by the vagus nerve and by nerve fibers from the celiac and superior mesenteric ganglia (see Figure 2-1). Many of the fibers within the vagus are preganglionic, whereas many from the abdominal ganglia are postganglionic. Some of the fibers within the vagus are cholinergic, whereas some from the abdominal plexuses are adrenergic. In addition, nerves that contain somatostatin, substance P, cholecystokinin (CCK), enkephalin, neuropeptide Y, and other transmitters have been identified in afferent and efferent vagal and splanchnic nerves. The exact pathways and physiologic roles of these nerves are being elucidated.

TYPES OF CONTRACTIONS

Between contractions, pressures within the lumen of the small intestine approximately equal the intraabdominal

FIGURE 5-1 ■ Intraluminal pressure changes recorded from the duodenum of a conscious human. Sensors placed 1 cm apart record changes in pressure that are phasic, lasting 4 to 5 seconds (s). Note that a rather large contraction can take place at one site while nothing is recorded 1 cm away on either side.

pressure. When the musculature contracts, the lumen is occluded partially or totally, and the pressure increases. Most contractions are local events and involve only 1 to 4 centimeters (cm) of bowel at a time. The contractions usually produce intraluminal pressure waves that appear as nearly symmetric peaks of uniform shape (Figure 5-1). In the human upper small bowel, contractions occur at any one site at multiple intervals of 5 seconds (Figure 5-2).

Occasionally other types of pressure waves can be recorded. One such type consists of an elevated baseline pressure that lasts from 10 seconds to 8 minutes. This wave seldom occurs alone and is usually accompanied by superimposed phasic changes in pressure.

The effect that any contraction has on the intestinal contents depends upon the state of the musculature above and below the point of the contraction. If a contraction is not coordinated with activity above and below, intestinal contents are displaced both proximally and distally during the contraction and may flow back during the period of relaxation. This would serve to mix and locally circulate the contents (Figure 5-3A). Such contractions appear to divide the bowel into segments, which accounts for the name given to this process—**segmentation**. If, however, the contractions at adjacent sites occur in a proximal-to-distal

sequence, aboral propulsion will result. (See video: http://www.wzw.tum.de/humanbiology/motvid01/movie_65_1mot01.wmv)

The small intestine is also capable of eliciting a highly coordinated contractile response that is propulsive in function. When an area of bowel is stimulated (e.g., by placement of a solid bolus of material in the lumen), the bowel responds with contraction orad and relaxation aborad to the point of stimulation. These events tend to move the material in an aboral direction (Figure 5-3B), and if they occur sequentially they can propel a bolus the entire length of the gut in a short time. This peristaltic response, first described by Bayliss and Starling, is known as the **law of the intestines**. Often it is invoked to explain how material is normally propelled through the small bowel. However, peristalsis involving long segments of intestine is seldom seen in normal persons, although peristaltic contractions involving short segments (1 to 4 cm) of intestine have been described.

PATTERNS OF CONTRACTIONS

Not only are there differences in individual contractions of the intestine, but there also are different patterns of

FIGURE 5-2 ■ Frequency distribution of 7572 contractions recorded at one site in the human small intestine. Note that the contractions are most frequent at multiples of 5 seconds (s), which is the approximate interval between slow waves in this region. *(From Christensen J, Glover JR, Macagno EO, et al: Statistics of contractions at a point in the human duodenum. Am J Physiol 221:1818-1823, 1971.)*

contractions. In fasting humans, contractions do not occur evenly over time. Rather, at each locus there are cycles consisting of phases of no or few contractions, followed by a phase of intense contractions (phase 3) that ends abruptly (Figure 5-4). The duration of each cycle is the same at adjacent loci of the bowel; however, the 5- to 10-minute phase of intense contractions does not occur simultaneously at all loci. Instead, this phase appears to migrate aborally, taking approximately 1.5 hours to sweep from the duodenum through the ileum. The characteristics of this pattern have earned it the title of **migrating motor complex** (MMC). This complex actually begins in the stomach (see Chapter 4). (See videos: http://www.wzw.tum.de/humanbiology/motvid02/movie_06_1mot02.wmv;http://www.wzw.tum.de/humanbiology/motvid02/movie_08_1mot02.wmv) Its functions appear to be to sweep undigested contents from the stomach, through the small intestine, and into the colon, and to maintain low bacterial counts in the upper intestine. MMCs cycle at intervals of about every 1.5 hours (Figure 5-5) as long as the person is fasting.

In nonfasting persons, contractions are spread more uniformly over time. In the human upper small bowel, contractions at any one site are present 14% to 34% of the recorded time, with the most common pattern being one to three sequential contractions separated by periods of 5, 10, 15, or 20 seconds. These contractions are of variable intensity, with none being as forceful as the intense contractions that occur during the MMC.

Contractions of the intestine are controlled by activities of the ICCs and smooth muscle cells, as well as by nerves and humoral substances. As in the stomach, smooth muscle cells in the small intestine have a membrane potential that fluctuates rhythmically with cyclic depolarizations and repolarizations of 5 to 15 millivolts (mV) (Figure 5-6). This **slow wave activity** (or basic electrical rhythm) is always present whether contractions are occurring or not. At any one site in the intestine, slow wave frequency is constant. Frequency, however, is not the same at all levels of the bowel. There is a decrease in frequency toward the ileocecal junction. In humans the frequency decreases from a mean of about 12 cycles/minute (cpm) in the duodenum to a mean of about 8 cpm in the terminal ileum. The decrease is not linear because frequency is constant throughout the duodenum and for about 10 cm into the jejunum. Beyond that point, frequency declines more or less linearly.

FIGURE 5-3 ■ The influence of contractions on contents within a region of intestine. Each panel depicts the region at three consecutive points in time. **A,** A contraction that is neither preceded by nor followed by other contractions serves to mix and locally circulate the intestinal contents. **B,** Contractions that have an orad-to-caudad sequence (left to right) serve to propel contents in a net aboral direction.

Although slow wave frequency is the same over the proximal small intestine, slow waves do not occur simultaneously at all points. Multiple electrodes detect a proximal-to-distal phase lag that simulates a propagated signal (see Figure 5-6).

In the small intestine, slow waves themselves do not initiate forceful contractions. Contractions are initiated by a second electrical event, often referred to as spike potential activity. **Spike potentials** are rapid depolarizations of the smooth muscle cell membrane that occur only during the depolarization phase of the slow wave. Because spike potentials are restricted to only one phase of the slow wave cycle, the contractions they initiate are phasic in nature. The muscle relaxes during the repolarization phase of the slow wave cycle.

During periods when every slow wave is accompanied by spike potentials, the intestine at any site contracts at the same frequency as the slow wave frequency

at that site. Thus slow wave frequency sets the maximum frequency of contractions at any one site. Also, because a gradient exists in the slow wave frequency along the small bowel, there is a gradient in the maximal frequency of contractions. For most of the time, however, spike potentials do not accompany every slow wave. During these periods, contractions at any one site occur at multiples of the slow wave interval. Thus it is no coincidence that in the human proximal bowel, slow waves occur every 5 seconds and contractions occur at multiple intervals of 5 seconds.

Although slow waves at adjacent sites along the bowel are always present and are temporally related, the occurrence of spike potentials is often localized. Thus sites 1 to 2 cm on either side of an area exhibiting slow waves with spike potentials may exhibit slow waves only. When this is the situation, segmenting contractions occur. On the other hand, when the occurrence of spike potentials is not localized, slow waves do influence the spatial relationships of contractions at adjacent sites. The phase lag in occurrence of slow waves at adjacent sites imposes a phase lag in the occurrence of contractions at adjacent sites.

As explained previously, not every slow wave is accompanied by spike potentials and muscle contraction. Occurrence of spike potentials and contractions is regulated by nervous activity and by circulating and locally released chemical agents. There are a number of reflexes that depend on the intrinsic neurons, the extrinsic neurons, or both. The **peristaltic reflex** (law of the intestines) described previously depends on an intact enteric nervous system. Application of neural blocking agents abolishes or greatly reduces this reflex. Another reflex, the **intestino-intestinal reflex,** depends on extrinsic neural connections. If an area of the bowel is grossly distended, contractile activity in the rest of the bowel is inhibited. Sectioning of the extrinsic nerves abolishes this reflex. Additionally, it is well known that changes in emotional state can induce alterations in small bowel motility. Thus the small bowel is under the influence of higher centers of the nervous system.

In addition to neural control, many circulating and endogenously released chemicals alter intestinal motility. Epinephrine released from the adrenal glands tends to inhibit contractions. Serotonin, which is contained in large quantities within the small intestine, stimulates contractions, as do certain of the prostaglandins.

FIGURE 5-4 ■ Contractions at three loci in the small bowel. Note that at each locus, phases of no or intermittent contractions are followed by a phase of continuous contractions that ends abruptly. Also note that the phase of continuous contractions appears to migrate aborally along the bowel. Such a pattern is called the migrating motor complex (MMC). min, minute; mm Hg, millimeters of mercury. *(From Rees WD, Malagelada JR, Miller H: Human interdigestive and postprandial gastrointestinal motor and gastrointestinal hormone patterns. Dig Dis Sci 27:321-329, 1982.)*

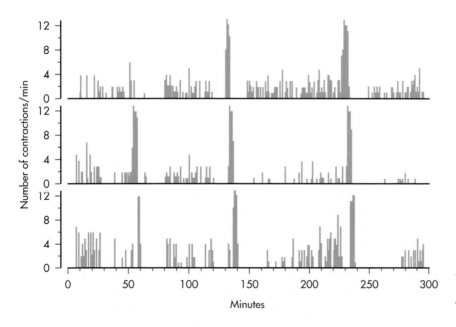

FIGURE 5-5 ■ Graphic presentation of the number of contractions at three loci in the small bowel. The number of contractions during each minute (min) of the recording was counted and plotted against the time of recording. The resulting histogram indicates cycles of activity at each locus. Note that MMCs recur at each locus at intervals of about 100 minutes and that the phases of intense contractions appear to migrate aborally. *(From Vantrappen G, Janssens J: The interdigestive motor complex of normal subjects and patients with bacterial overgrowth of the small intestine. J Clin Invest 59:1158-1166, 1977.)*

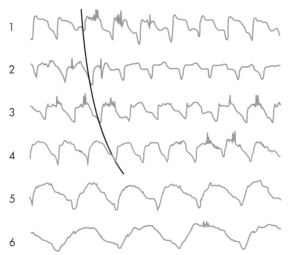

FIGURE 5-6 ■ Slow waves and spike potentials from multiple sites in the small intestine. Tracings 1 to 6 illustrate activity from progressively distal areas. The solid line connecting the slow waves in tracings 1 to 4 denotes the apparent propagation in the region of a slow wave frequency plateau. Tracings 5 and 6 show decreases in slow wave frequency at more distal areas. The rapid transients that occur on the peaks of some of the slow waves represent spike potentials.

Several hormones also alter intestinal motility. Gastrin, CCK, motilin, and insulin tend to stimulate contractions, whereas secretin and glucagon tend to inhibit them. The exact role of these chemical agents in the regulation of motility is yet to be clarified.

The presence of a characteristic pattern of contractions during fasting—the MMC—indicates complex controlling mechanisms. The hormone motilin may be involved in regulating MMC cycle length. Plasma levels of motilin fluctuate with the same periodicity as for the phase of intense duodenal contractions, and exogenously administered motilin will initiate a premature MMC. Enteric nerves also are involved, because their disruption alters MMC initiation and migration. Extrinsic nerves do not seem to be required. Segments of intestine that have been extrinsically denervated still exhibit MMCs. However, extrinsic neural activity can modify characteristics of the MMC.

Feeding abolishes MMCs and institutes a pattern of more or less continuous contractions of varying amplitude. The change in pattern caused by feeding probably is brought about by hormones such as gastrin and CCK, which are released during feeding, and by neural mechanisms.

CLINICAL APPLICATIONS

Primary disorders of small intestine motility are rare. The small intestine may be involved in certain general disorders of smooth muscle of the gastrointestinal (GI) and urinary tracts. The cause of these disorders is unknown, but in some patients there may be a genetic basis. When the disorder is clinically apparent, a patient will appear to have episodes of intestinal obstruction; however, the problem seems to involve a failure of propulsive motility rather than an obstruction. Thus the name **idiopathic pseudo-obstruction** has been coined. In some patients with this syndrome, the smooth muscle cells and ICCs are involved. In other patients, histologic studies show changes in enteric nerves.

Altered small intestinal motility resulting in delayed transit frequently accompanies a variety of diseases and clinical conditions. Perhaps the most common is the transient ileus or apparent paralysis of the small intestine sometimes seen after abdominal surgery. However, intra-abdominal inflammation (e.g., pancreatitis, appendicitis, abscess) may produce a similar picture. Systemic diseases such as diabetes mellitus and amyloidosis, metabolic alterations such as potassium depletion, and administration of drugs, particularly anticholinergics, all may have an adverse effect on intestinal transit. Mixing probably is impaired as well, although this is less clinically apparent.

Alternatively, rapid intestinal transit is seen in certain malabsorptive states induced by infectious agents, allergic reaction, and various pharmacologic agents. In these conditions both motility and absorption are affected. In most disease states it is not clear whether changes in motility are primary (caused by the disease) or secondary (caused by the presence of unabsorbed or secreted material).

CLINICAL TESTS

Auscultation to detect "bowel sounds" probably is the most common means used to assess bowel activity. In addition, observing the movement of barium by x-ray and of isotopes by scintigraphy (see Chapter 4) can yield some information on transit time through the small bowel. Unfortunately, these methods are not precise. Advances in technology have made the recording of intraluminal pressures rather easy in normal persons and patients with minimal GI dysfunction. However, the inaccessibility of the small intestine and the difficulty in placing intraluminal sensors in patients with major dysmotility limit the routine use of direct recordings of intestinal contractions as a diagnostic tool.

SUMMARY

1. Movement of contents within the intestinal lumen depends on the type of contraction. Segmenting contractions cause mixing and local circulation of contents. Peristaltic contractions cause net aboral transit.

2. During digestion of a meal, most contractions are of the segmenting type, with short peristaltic contractions occurring randomly. During interdigestive periods, bursts of intense peristaltic contractions envelop each region of the intestine about every 90 minutes. Each burst appears to begin in the stomach and migrate aborally along the intestine such that it reaches the terminal ileum in about 90 minutes. This activity is called the MMC.

3. Intestinal slow waves are cyclic depolarizations and repolarizations of muscle cell membranes. At any locus of the intestine, slow waves are present at a constant frequency (i.e., around 12 per minute in the duodenum and 8 per minute in the ileum). At adjacent loci, slow waves appear to propagate aborally.

4. Spike potentials are rapid fluctuations in membrane potential that are superimposed on the depolarization phase of the slow wave. They, not the slow waves themselves, initiate contractions of the muscle. Spike potentials do not accompany every slow wave. Their presence and pattern depend on the digestive state and on neural and humoral activities.

5. Enteric nerves coordinate both the type and patterns of contraction. The phase of intense contractions of the MMC in the upper intestine may be initiated by the release of motilin. The conversion of the MMC pattern to the digestive pattern may be due in part to the release of hormones such as gastrin and CCK.

KEY WORDS AND CONCEPTS

- Myenteric/Auerbach plexus
- Segmentation
- Law of the intestines
- Migrating motor complex
- Slow wave activity
- Spike potentials
- Peristaltic reflex
- Intestino-intestinal reflex
- Idiopathic pseudo-obstruction

REFERENCES

Hasler WL: Small intestinal motility. In Johnson LR (ed): Physiology of the Gastrointestinal Tract, vol 1, 4th ed. San Diego, Elsevier, 2006.

Weisbrodt NW: Motility of the small intestine. In Johnson LR (ed): Physiology of the Gastrointestinal Tract, 2nd ed. New York, Raven Press, 1987.

Wingate DL: Backward and forward with the migrating complex. Dig Dis Sci 26:641-666, 1981.

6

MOTILITY OF THE LARGE INTESTINE

NORMAN W. WEISBRODT

Contractions of the large intestine are organized to allow for optimal absorption of water and electrolytes, net aboral movement of contents, and storage and orderly evacuation of feces.

ANATOMIC CONSIDERATIONS

Anatomically the human large intestine is divided into the **cecum;** the **ascending, transverse, descending**, and **sigmoid colon;** the **rectum;** and the **anal canal**. The muscular layers of the large intestine are composed of both longitudinally and circularly arranged fibers. Longitudinal fibers are concentrated into three flat bands called the **taeniae coli**. These run from the cecum to the rectum, where the fibers fan out to form a more continuous longitudinal coat. The circular layer of muscle fibers is continuous from the cecum to the anal canal, where it increases in thickness to form the **internal anal sphincter**. Overlapping and slightly distal to the internal anal sphincter are layers of striated muscle. These striated muscle bundles make up the **external anal sphincter**.

In humans the external features of the large intestine differ from those of the small intestine. In addition to the presence of taeniae coli, the colon appears to be divided into segments called **haustra** or **haustrations** (Figure 6-1). Haustra probably are the result of structural and functional properties of the colon. Points of concentration of muscular tissue and mucosal foldings can be found in colons examined post mortem.

Also, haustra are more prominent in areas of the colon that possess taeniae coli. Haustra are not fixed, however. Segmental colonic contractions appear, disappear, and re-form at another locus. Thus haustral formation also has a dynamic component because of the contractile activity of colonic musculature.

The large intestine, like other areas of the bowel, is innervated by the autonomic nervous system (ANS). The enteric system consists partly of many nerve cell bodies and endings that lie between the circular and the longitudinal muscle coats. In areas of the large intestine with taeniae, this myenteric plexus is concentrated beneath them. Cells of the myenteric plexus receive input from a variety of receptors within the intestine, as well as by way of the extrinsic nerves. Axons from these cells innervate the muscle layers. Extrinsic innervation to the large intestine comes from both parasympathetic and sympathetic branches of the ANS. There are two pathways of parasympathetic innervation: the cecum and the ascending and transverse portions of the colon are innervated by the vagus nerve; the descending and sigmoid areas of the colon and the rectum are innervated by pelvic nerves from the sacral region of the spinal cord. The pelvic nerves enter the colon near the rectosigmoid junction and project orally and aborally within the plane of the myenteric plexus. These projections, called **shunt fascicles,** innervate myenteric nerves en route. The vagus and pelvic nerves consist primarily of preganglionic efferent fibers and

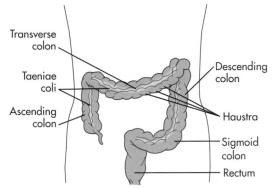

FIGURE 6-1 ■ Anatomy of the colon. The colon is shorter and of larger diameter than the small intestine. The longitudinal smooth muscle is concentrated into three bands (taeniae coli) in all regions except the rectum. Note that all regions except the rectum possess haustra. The exact cause of haustration is not known. They are formed partly by contractions of the circular muscle; however, because they are still present after death, some investigators believe they have a permanent structural basis.

many afferent fibers. The efferent fibers supposedly synapse with the nerve cell bodies of the myenteric and other intrinsic plexuses. The proximal regions of the large intestine are sympathetically innervated by fibers that come from the superior mesenteric ganglion. More distal regions receive input from the inferior mesenteric ganglion. The distal rectum and anal canal are innervated by sympathetic fibers from the hypogastric plexus. Most of the sympathetic fibers are

postganglionic efferent and afferent fibers. The external anal sphincter, a striated muscle, is innervated by the somatic pudendal nerves.

As in other regions of the gut, a number of diverse chemicals serve as mediators at presynaptic and post-synaptic junctions within the autonomic innervation to the large intestine. Acetylcholine (ACh) and tachykinins such as substance P serve as major excitatory mediators, and nitric oxide (NO), vasoactive intestinal peptide (VIP), and possibly adenosine triphosphate (ATP) serve as major inhibitory mediators. Transmission between the pudendal nerves and the external anal sphincter is mediated by ACh.

CONTRACTIONS OF THE CECUM AND ASCENDING COLON

The flow of contents from the small intestine into the large intestine is intermittent and regulated partly by a sphincteric mechanism at the **ileocecal junction**. A sensor placed in the junction records pressures that are several millimeters of mercury (mm Hg) greater than those in the ileum or colon. The pressure, however, is not constant, for the sphincter relaxes periodically; during this time ileal contractions propel contents into the large intestine (Figure 6-2A). Once material reaches the proximal large intestine, it is acted on by a wide variety of contractions. A majority of these are segmental in nature, with durations of 12 to 60 seconds. The pressures generated by these contractions vary in amplitude, ranging between about 10 and 50 mm Hg.

FIGURE 6-2 ■ Intraluminal pressures recorded at the level of the ileocecal sphincter. Note that a resting pressure of 20 to 40 mm Hg exists. **A,** Distention of the ileum causes sphincteric relaxation and thus allows flow of contents from the ileum into the colon. **B,** Distention of the colon, by contrast, causes contraction of the sphincter to prevent passage of contents from the colon to the ileum. *(From Cohen S, Harris LD, Levitan R: Manometric characteristics of the human ileocecal junctional zone, Gastroenterology 54:72-75, 1968.)*

It is believed that these contractions are partly responsible for the haustrations seen in the colon. At adjacent sites, contractions usually occur independently. Thus, they slowly move the contents back and forth, mixing and exposing them to the mucosa for absorption of water and electrolytes. In addition to pressure changes caused by segmental contractions, a large variety of other pressure waves have been recorded. Attempts to classify these have been made, but the degree of overlap of pressure profiles makes classification difficult.

Occasionally, segmental contractions are organized in an oral-to-aboral direction; thus propulsion over short distances takes place. Usually, however, propulsion occurs during a characteristic sequence termed **mass movement**. Segmental activity suddenly ceases, and along with its disappearance there is a loss of haustrations. The colon then undergoes a contraction that sweeps intraluminal contents in an aboral direction (Figure 6-3A to C). After the mass movement, haustrations and phasic contractions return (Figure 6-3D). Mass movements are infrequent in healthy people and are estimated to occur only one to three times daily. Because they are such infrequent events, they have not been studied in any great detail in normal persons.

CONTRACTIONS OF THE DESCENDING AND SIGMOID COLON

By the time material reaches the descending and sigmoid colon, it has changed from a liquid to a semisolid state. Although there is less absorption of water and electrolytes from these portions of the colon, motility studies have demonstrated that contractions of the

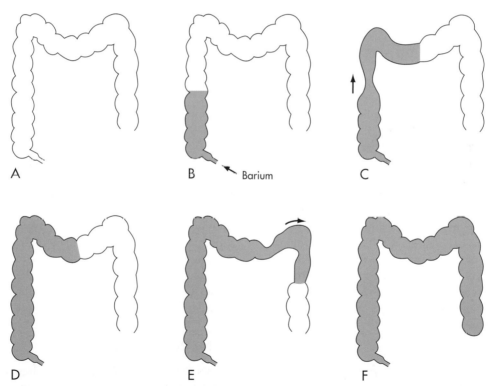

FIGURE 6-3 ■ Two mass movements. **A,** Appearance of the colon before the entry of barium sulfate. **B,** As the barium enters from the ileum, it is acted on by haustral contractions. **C,** As more barium enters, a portion is swept into and through an area of the colon that has lost its haustral markings. **D,** The barium is acted on by the returning haustral contractions. **E,** A second mass movement propels the barium into and through areas of the transverse and descending colon. **F,** Haustrations again return. This type of contraction accomplishes most of the movement of feces through the colon.

segmenting type are more frequent here than in the ascending and transverse colon. These segmenting contractions do not result in propulsion. On the contrary, they offer resistance and thus retard the flow of contents from more proximal regions into the rectum. Propulsion into and through these areas probably also occurs during mass movements. Here too there is a loss of segmental activity and the haustrations that precede transport (Figure 6-3E and F). Thus material that enters these regions during a mass movement is acted on to further reduce its liquid content and is then propelled into the rectum during a subsequent mass movement.

MOTILITY OF THE RECTUM AND ANAL CANAL

The rectum usually is empty or nearly so. Although very little material is present, contractions do occur in this region. In fact, the upper regions of the rectum contract segmentally more frequently than does the sigmoid colon. This activity tends to retard the flow of contents into the rectum. When the rectum fills, it does so intermittently. During a mass movement or during an aborally directed sequence of segmental contractions of the sigmoid colon, some material passes into the rectum.

Normally the anal canal is closed because of contraction of the internal anal sphincter. When the rectum is distended by fecal material, however, the internal sphincter relaxes as part of the **rectosphincteric reflex** (Figure 6-4). Rectal distention also elicits a sensation that signals the urge for defecation. If environmental conditions are not conducive to defecation, voluntary contractions of the external sphincter can overcome the reflex. Relaxation of the internal sphincter is transient because the receptors within the rectal wall accommodate the stimulus of distention. Thus the internal anal sphincter regains its tone, and the sensation subsides until the passage of more contents into the rectum. The rectum can accommodate rather large quantities of material, so it acts as a storage organ.

If the rectosphincteric reflex is elicited at a time when evacuation is convenient, defecation occurs. **Defecation** is accomplished by a series of voluntary and involuntary acts. When rectal distention is followed by defecation, muscles of the descending and sigmoid colon and

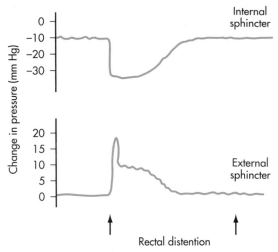

FIGURE 6-4 ■ Intraluminal pressure recorded at the level of the internal and external anal sphincters. Rectal distention causes relaxation of the internal sphincter and contraction of the external sphincter. Note, however, that the changes in sphincteric pressures are transient even though rectal distention is maintained. This is related to the accommodation of the stretch receptors within the wall of the rectum. (Modified from Schuster MM, Hookman P, Hendrix TR: Simultaneous manometric recording of internal and external anal sphincteric reflexes. Johns Hopkins Med J 116: 70-88, 1965.)

the rectum may contract to propel contents toward the anal canal. Then both internal and external sphincters relax to allow passage of the bolus. Normally these events are accompanied by voluntary acts that raise intra-abdominal pressure and lower the pelvic floor. Intra-abdominal pressure is increased by contractions of the diaphragm and musculature of the abdominal wall. Simultaneously the musculature of the pelvic floor relaxes to allow the increased abdominal pressure to force the floor downward.

CONTROL OF MOTILITY

Factors that control motility of the large intestine are complex and poorly understood. As in the stomach and small intestine, motility in the large intestine is influenced by at least four factors: interstitial cells of Cajal–smooth muscle properties, enteric nerves, extrinsic nerves, and circulating or locally released chemicals.

The tone of the ileocecal sphincter is basically myogenic. It is modified, however, by nervous and humoral factors. Distention of the colon causes an increase in sphincteric tension, a reflex probably mediated via the enteric nerves (see Figure 6-2B). Distention of the ileum causes relaxation, also probably mediated via the enteric nerves (see Figure 6-2A). Relaxation of the sphincter and an increase in the contractile activity of the ileum occur with or shortly after eating. This has been termed the **gastroileal reflex**. One view is that the reflex is mediated by the gastrointestinal (GI) hormones, primarily gastrin and cholecystokinin (CCK). Both of these hormones cause an increase in the contractile activity of the ileum, as well as a relaxation of the ileocecal sphincter. Some investigators, however, think that this reflex is mediated via the extrinsic autonomic nerves to the intestine.

Smooth muscle cells of the ascending, transverse, descending, and sigmoid colon, and of the rectum, exhibit fluctuations in their membrane potential. Cyclic depolarizations and repolarizations that possess some of the characteristics of small intestinal slow waves can be recorded. As in the small intestine, these slow waves are thought to depend on interactions between smooth muscle cells and interstitial cells of Cajal. Potential changes that resemble spike potentials also are recorded. These probably initiate contractions, but the exact relationships between changes in potential and contractile activity have not been clarified. In addition, investigators have recorded various oscillations in membrane potential that fit descriptions of neither slow wave nor spike potential activities. Their origin and function are less clear.

Enteric neurons probably are involved in the control of colonic contractions. A peristaltic reflex can be initiated in the colon, and this reflex is mediated by nerve elements within the myenteric plexus. These plexal nerves seem to be predominantly inhibitory because in their absence the colon is contracted tonically. A number of colonic reflexes have their pathways in the extrinsic nerves. Distention of remote areas of the bowel induces an inhibition of contractions. The pathway for this reflex includes the inferior mesenteric ganglion and also may include the spinal cord. In addition, several investigations have demonstrated that emotional state has a marked influence on colonic motility. These influences of the central nervous system are mediated by the extrinsic nerves.

The GI hormones, as well as epinephrine and the prostaglandins, affect colonic motility. Gastrin and CCK cause increases in colonic activity and have been implicated in the mass movement that sometimes is seen after eating. Epinephrine causes inhibition of all contractile activity, whereas the prostaglandins (primarily E type) cause a decrease in segmenting contractions and an increase in propulsive activity. The importance of these agents in regulating colonic motility is not known.

The rectosphincteric reflex and the act of defecation are under neural control. Part of the control lies in the enteric nervous system. The reflex, however, is reinforced by activity of neurons within the spinal cord. Destruction of the nerves to the anorectal area can result in fecal retention. The sensation of rectal distention, as well as voluntary control of the external anal sphincter, is mediated by pathways within the spinal cord that lead to the cerebral cortex. Destruction of these pathways leads to a loss of voluntary control of defecation.

CLINICAL SIGNIFICANCE

Abnormal transit of material through the colon is common. Delayed transit leads to **constipation**; in most situations, however, this is dietary in origin. There is a direct correlation among increased dietary fiber, increased colonic intraluminal bulk, and enhanced transit through the colon. How motility of the colon contributes to these changes in transit is not known. A particularly interesting and dramatic clinical disorder in which severe constipation is seen is congenital megacolon (**Hirschsprung's disease**), which is characterized by an absence of the enteric nervous system in the distal colon. The internal anal sphincter is always involved, and often the disease extends proximally into the rectum. The involved segment exhibits increased tone, has a very narrow lumen, and is devoid of propulsive activity. As a result, the colon proximal to the diseased segment becomes dilated, thus producing a megacolon. This condition is treated through surgical removal of the diseased segment.

In adults, the most common GI disorder for which medical advice is sought is **irritable bowel syndrome**. This disorder gives rise most often to abdominal pain and altered bowel habit (constipation and/or diarrhea). In limited observations, exaggerated segmental contractions in the sigmoid colon have been seen, particularly in response to stimulants such as morphine. During stress, patients with irritable bowel syndrome and constipation exhibit increased segmentation in the sigmoid colon, whereas those with diarrhea exhibit decreased segmentation. In addition to motility disorders, sensory hypersensitivity to visceral stimulation may play a role. The cause of this disorder remains unknown. One theory suggests that altered motility may reflect the conditioning of autonomic responses from repeated exposure to stressful situations. Another suggests that gastrointestinal infections and alterations in normal colonic flora play a role in the etiology of irritable bowel syndrome.

In older age groups, **diverticula** (outpouchings of mucosa that extend through the muscular wall) frequently develop in the colon. There is evidence to suggest that abnormal colonic motility leads to diverticulum formation because of the generation of increased intraluminal pressure. However, a direct correlation among abnormal motility, symptoms, and the presence of diverticula cannot always be demonstrated.

CLINICAL TESTS

Despite the large numbers of patients in whom disordered colonic motility is suspected, techniques for monitoring contractions are not in general clinical use. Most often, radiologic procedures are used to provide limited information. In one test, radiopaque markers are ingested daily for 3 days. On the fourth day, a radiograph is taken and the number of markers in each region of the colon is noted and compared with normal values. Measurements of intraluminal pressures and myoelectric activity are feasible, especially in the sigmoid colon and rectum because these areas are readily accessible. To date, such techniques are mainly used in investigative studies.

The behavior of both the internal and the external anal sphincters, and the response to rectal distention, can be measured by the careful placement of two small intraluminal balloons in the anal canal. A third balloon is placed in the rectum and distended to monitor the components of the defecation reflex. This technique has usefulness for patients with suspected neurologic disorders that result in impaired defecation.

S U M M A R Y

1. The muscular anatomy of the colon is characterized by concentration of the longitudinal muscle into bands called taeniae coli. Contraction of the taeniae coli and the circular muscle results in haustrations.

2. A majority of colonic contractions are of the segmenting type, which aid in the absorption of water and electrolytes. The frequency of segmenting contractions is higher in the descending and sigmoid colon than in areas located more orad. This retards aboral progression.

3. Aboral movement of contents is slow, usually taking days to pass material through the colon. Most aboral movement takes place during infrequent peristaltic contractions called mass movements.

4. Tonic contraction of the internal anal sphincter maintains closure of the anal canal. Distention of the rectum elicits relaxation of the internal anal

sphincter and causes the urge to defecate. Defecation can be prevented by voluntary contraction of the external anal sphincter while the rectum accommodates to the distention and the internal anal sphincter regains its tone. Relaxation of the external anal sphincter during this time leads to defecation.

5. Colonic slow waves are cyclic depolarizations and repolarizations of muscle cell membranes that appear to set the timing of segmental contractions. Neural activity and hormone levels influence the intensity of segmental contractions.

6. Mass movements are regulated by activities of the intrinsic and extrinsic nerves and possibly by the hormones gastrin and CCK. The rectosphincteric reflex is regulated by intrinsic, extrinsic autonomic, and somatic nerves.

KEY WORDS AND CONCEPTS

- Cecum
- Ascending/transverse/descending/sigmoid colon
- Rectum
- Anal canal
- Taeniae coli
- Internal anal sphincter
- External anal sphincter
- Haustra/haustrations
- Shunt fascicles
- Ileocecal junction
- Mass movement
- Rectosphincteric reflex
- Defecation
- Gastroileal reflex
- Constipation
- Hirschsprung's disease
- Irritable bowel syndrome
- Diverticula

REFERENCES

Christensen J: The motility of the colon. In Johnson LR (ed): Physiology of the Gastrointestinal Tract, vol 1, 3rd ed. New York, Raven Press, 1994.

Phillips SF: Motility disorders of the colon. In Yamada T, Alpers DH, Laine L, et al (eds): Textbook of gastroenterology, vol 1, 3rd ed. Philadelphia, Lippincott Williams & Wilkins, 1999.

Sarna S: Large intestinal motility. In Johnson LR (ed): Physiology of the Gastrointestinal Tract, 4th ed. San Diego, Elsevier, 2006.

7

SALIVARY SECRETION

LEONARD R. JOHNSON

Although the salivary glands are not essential to life, their secretions are important for the hygiene and comfort of the mouth and teeth. The functions of saliva may be divided into those concerned with **lubrication, protection,** and **digestion.** An active process produces saliva in large quantities relative to the weight of the salivary glands. Saliva is hyposmotic at all rates of secretion, and in contrast with the other gastrointestinal (GI) secretions, the rate of secretion is almost totally under the control of the nervous system. Another characteristic of this regulation is that both branches of the autonomic nervous system (ANS) stimulate secretion. However, the parasympathetic system provides a much greater stimulus than that due to the sympathetic system.

FUNCTIONS OF SALIVA

The lubricating ability of saliva depends primarily on its content of **mucus.** In the mouth, mixing saliva with food lubricates the ingested material and facilitates the swallowing process. The lubricating effect of saliva is also necessary for speech, as evidenced by the glass of water normally found on the podium of a public speaker.

Saliva exerts its effects through a variety of different mechanisms. It protects the mouth by buffering and diluting noxious substances. Hot solutions of tea, coffee, or soup, for example, are diluted and cooled by saliva. Foul-tasting substances can be washed from the mouth by copious salivation. Similarly, the salivary glands are stimulated strongly before vomiting. The corrosive gastric acid and pepsin that are brought up into the esophagus and mouth are thereby neutralized and diluted by saliva. Dry mouth, or xerostomia, is associated with chronic infections of the buccal mucosa and with dental caries. Saliva dissolves and washes out food particles from between the teeth. A number of specialized constituents of saliva have antibacterial actions. These include a **lysozyme,** which attacks bacterial cell walls; **lactoferrin,** which chelates iron, preventing the multiplication of organisms that require it for growth; and the **binding glycoprotein for immunoglobulin A (IgA),** which in combination with IgA forms secretory IgA that in turn is immunologically active against viruses and bacteria. Various inorganic compounds are taken up by the salivary glands, concentrated, and secreted in saliva. These include fluoride and calcium, which are subsequently incorporated into the teeth.

The contributions made by saliva to normal digestion include dissolving and washing away food particles on the taste buds to enable one to taste the next morsel of food eaten. Saliva contains two enzymes, one directed toward carbohydrates and the other toward fat. An α-**amylase** called **ptyalin** cleaves internal α-1,4-glycosidic bonds present in starch. Exhaustive digestion of starch by this enzyme, which is identical to pancreatic amylase, produces maltose, maltotriose, and α-limit dextrins, which contain the α-1,6 branch points of the original molecule. Salivary amylase has a pH optimum of 7, and it is rapidly denatured at pH 4. However, because a large portion of a meal often remains unmixed for a considerable length of time in the orad stomach, the salivary enzyme may account for the digestion of as much as 75% of the starch present before it is denatured by gastric acid. In the absence of salivary amylase there is no defect in carbohydrate digestion, for the pancreatic enzyme is secreted in amounts sufficient to digest all of the starch present.

The serous salivary glands of the tongue secrete the second digestive enzyme, **lingual lipase,** which plays a role in the hydrolysis of dietary lipid. Unlike pancreatic lipase, its properties allow it to act in all parts of the upper GI tract. Thus the ability of lingual lipase to hydrolyze lipids is not affected by surface-active detergents such as bile salts, medium-chain fatty acids, and lecithin. It has an acidic pH optimum and remains active through the stomach and into the intestine.

ANATOMY AND INNERVATION OF THE SALIVARY GLANDS

The salivary glands are a collection of somewhat dissimilar structures in the mouth that produce a common juice (the saliva), although the composition of the secretion from different salivary glands differs. The largest of the salivary structures are the paired **parotid glands,**

located near the angle of the jaw and the ear. They secrete a fairly watery juice, whereas the smaller bilateral **submandibular** and **sublingual glands** elaborate a more viscid saliva. Other, still smaller glands are present in the mucosa covering the palate, buccal areas, lips, and tongue.

Most of the salivary glands are ectodermal in origin. The combined secretion of the parotid and submandibular glands constitutes 90% of the volume of saliva, which in a normal adult amounts to a half liter daily. The specific gravity of this mixed juice ranges from 1.000 to 1.010.

The microscopic structure of the salivary glands combines many features observed in another exocrine gland, the pancreas. A salivary gland consists of a blind-end system of microscopic ducts that branch out from grossly visible ducts. One main duct opens into the mouth from each gland. The functional unit of the salivary duct system, the **salivon,** is depicted in Figure 7-1. At the blind end is the **acinus,** surrounded by polygonal acinar cells. These cells secrete the initial saliva, including water, electrolytes, and organic molecules such as amylase. Sodium and water follow the chloride. Subsequently, the solutes and fluid diffuse out of the acinar cell into the duct lumen to form the

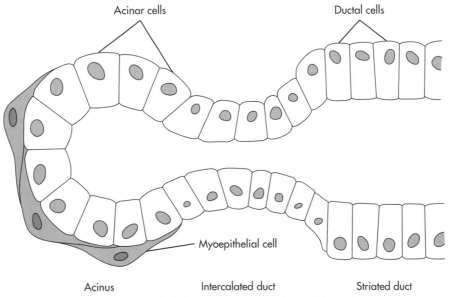

FIGURE 7-1 ■ Cells lining the various portions of the salivon.

initial saliva. The acinar cells are surrounded, in turn, by **myoepithelial cells.** The myoepithelial cells rest upon the basement membrane of acinar cells. They contain an actinomycin and have motile extensions. The next segment of the salivon is the **intercalated duct**, which may be associated with additional myoepithelial cells. Contraction of myoepithelial cells serves to expel formed saliva from the acinus, oppose retrograde movement of the juice during active secretion of saliva, shorten and widen the internal diameter of the intercalated duct (thereby lowering resistance to the flowing saliva), and prevent distention of the acinus (distention of the blind end of the salivon would permit back-diffusion of formed saliva through the stretched surface of the acinus). Thus, the myoepithelial cells support the acinus against the increased intraluminal pressures that occur during secretion.

Whenever there is an abrupt need for saliva in the mouth (e.g., immediately before vomiting), myoepithelial cell contraction propels the secretion into the main duct of the gland. Other exocrine glands, such as the mammary glands and the pancreas, also possess myoepithelial cells.

The intercalated duct soon widens to become the **striated duct,** lined by columnar epithelial cells that resemble the epithelial components of the renal tubule in both shape and function. The saliva in the intercalated duct is similar in ionic composition to plasma. Changes from that composition occur because of ion exchanges in the striated duct. As saliva traverses the striated duct, sodium is actively reabsorbed from the juice, and potassium is transported into it. Calcium also enters secreting duct cells during salivation. Similarly, there is anionic exchange, with chloride being reabsorbed from the saliva and bicarbonate being added to it.

The striated duct epithelium is considered to be a fairly "tight" sheet membrane. That is, its surface is fairly impermeable to the back-diffusion of water from the saliva into the tissue, and osmotic gradients develop between the saliva and interstitial fluid through the reabsorption of sodium and chloride, which results in a hypotonic saliva.

The blood supplied to the salivary glands is distributed by branches of the external carotid artery. The direction of arterial flow within the substance of each salivary gland is opposite the direction of flowing

saliva within the ducts of each salivon. The arterioles break up into capillaries around the acini, as well as in nonacinar areas. Blood from nonacinar areas passes through portal venules back to the acinar capillaries, from which a second set of venules then drain all the blood to the systemic venous circulation. The rate of blood flow through resting salivary tissue is approximately 20 times that through muscle. This in part accounts for the prodigious amounts of saliva produced relative to the weight of the glands.

Both components of the ANS reach the salivary glands. The parasympathetic preganglionic fibers are delivered by the facial and glossopharyngeal nerves to autonomic ganglia, from which the postganglionic fibers pass to individual glands. The sympathetic preganglionic nerves originate at the cervical ganglion, whose postganglionic fibers extend to the glands in the periarterial spaces (these relationships appear in Figure 7-2). Parasympathetic and sympathetic mediators regulate all known salivary gland functions to an extraordinary degree. Their influence includes major effects upon not only secretion but also blood flow, ductular smooth muscle activity, growth, and metabolism of the salivary glands.

COMPOSITION OF SALIVA

The major constituents of saliva are water, electrolytes, and a few enzymes. The **unique properties** of this GI juice are (1) its large volume relative to the mass of glands that secrete saliva, (2) its low osmolality, (3) its high potassium concentration, and (4) the specific organic materials it contains.

Inorganic Composition

Compared with other secretory organs of the GI tract, the salivary glands elaborate a remarkably large volume of juice per gram (g) of tissue. Thus, for example, an entire pancreas may reach a maximal rate of secretion of 1 milliliter (mL)/minute, whereas at the highest rates of secretion in some animals, a tiny submaxillary gland can secrete 1 mL/g/minute, a 50-fold higher rate. In humans, the salivary glands secrete at rates several-fold higher than other GI organs per unit weight of tissue.

The osmolality of saliva is significantly lower than that of plasma at all but the highest rates of secretion,

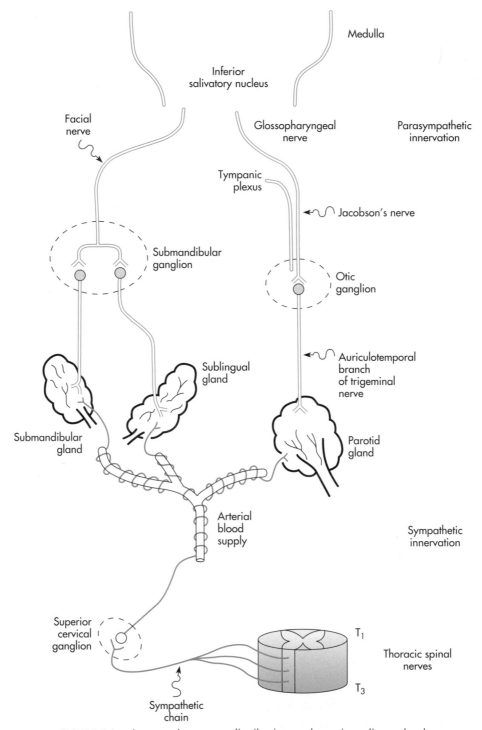

FIGURE 7-2 ■ Autonomic nervous distribution to the major salivary glands.

FIGURE 7-3 ■ Concentrations of major ions in the saliva as a function of the rate of salivary secretion. Values in plasma are shown for comparison.

when the saliva becomes isotonic with plasma. As the secretory rate of the salivon increases, the osmolality of its saliva also increases.

The concentrations of electrolytes in saliva vary with the rate of secretion (Figure 7-3). The potassium concentration of saliva is 2 to 30 times that of the plasma, depending on the rate of secretion, the nature of the stimulus, the plasma potassium concentration, and the level of mineralocorticoids in the circulation. Saliva has the highest potassium concentration of any digestive juice; maximal concentration values approach those within cells. These remarkable levels of salivary potassium imply the existence of an energy-dependent transport mechanism within the salivon. In most species the concentration of Na^+ in saliva is always less than that in plasma, and, as the secretory rate increases, the Na^+ concentration also increases. In general, Cl^- concentrations parallel those of Na^+. These findings suggest that Na^+ and Cl^- are secreted and then reabsorbed as the saliva passes through the ducts. The concentration of HCO_3^- in saliva is higher than that in plasma, except at low flow rates. This also accounts for the changes in the pH of saliva. At basal rates of flow the pH is slightly acidic but rapidly rises to around 8 as flow is stimulated. The relationships between ion concentrations and flow rates (shown in Figure 7-3) vary somewhat depending on the stimulus.

The relationships shown in Figure 7-3 are explained by two basic types of studies that indicate how the final saliva is produced. First, fluid collected by micropuncture of the intercalated ducts contains Na^+, K^+, Cl^-, and HCO_3^- in concentrations approximately equal to their plasma concentrations. This fluid also is isotonic to plasma. Second, if one perfuses a salivary gland duct with fluid containing ions in concentrations similar to those of plasma, Na^+ and Cl^- concentrations are decreased and the K^+ and HCO_3^- concentrations are increased when the fluid is collected at the duct opening. The fluid also becomes hypotonic, and the longer the fluid remains in the duct (i.e., the slower the rate of perfusion) the greater the changes. These data indicate, first, that the acini secrete a fluid similar to plasma in its concentration of ions, and, second, that as the fluid moves down the duct, Na^+ and Cl^- are reabsorbed and K^+ and HCO_3^- are secreted into the saliva. The higher the flow of saliva, the less time is available for modification, and the final saliva more closely resembles plasma in its ionic makeup (see Figure 7-3). At low flow rates K^+ increases considerably, and Na^+ and Cl^- decrease. Because most salivary agonists stimulate HCO_3^- secretion, the HCO_3^- concentration remains relatively high, even at high rates of secretion. Some K^+ and HCO_3^- are reabsorbed in exchange for Na^+ and Cl^-, but much more Na^+ and

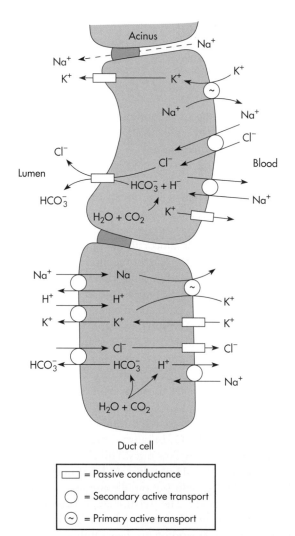

FIGURE 7-4 ■ Movements of ions and water in the acinus and duct of the salivon.

Cl^- leave the duct, causing the saliva to become hypotonic. Because the duct epithelium is relatively impermeable to water, the final product remains hypotonic. These processes are depicted in Figure 7-4.

Current evidence indicates that Cl^- is the primary ion that is actively secreted by the acinar cells (Figure 7-5). No evidence exists for direct active secretion of Na^+. The secretory mechanism for Cl^- is inhibited by ouabain, indicating that it depends on the Na^+-K^+ pump in the basolateral membrane. The active pumping of Na^+ out of the cell creates a diffusion gradient for Na^+ to enter across the basolateral membrane. Cl^- is cotransported with Na^+ into the cell to preserve electrical neutrality. This increases the electrochemical potential of Cl^- within the cell, and Cl^- diffuses down this gradient into the lumen via an electrogenic ion channel that also allows HCO_3^- to enter the lumen. The secretion of HCO_3^- is facilitated by the movement of H^+ out of the cell in exchange for Na^+. Na^+ moves paracellularly through the tight junctions and into the lumen, preserving electroneutrality; water follows down its osmotic gradient. There is now evidence for a Ca^{++}-activated K^+ channel in the basolateral membrane. Exodus of K^+ increases the electronegativity of the cytosol, increasing the driving force for the entry of Cl^- and HCO_3^- into the lumen. Agents that stimulate salivary secretion increase the activity of all these channels and transport processes.

Within the ducts (see Figure 7-5), Na^+ is actively absorbed and K^+ is actively secreted. These processes depend on several transporters that are powered by the Na^+ gradient created by the Na^+,K^+-adenosine triphosphatase (ATPase) in the basolateral membrane. The apical membrane contains Na^+-H^+ and Cl^--HCO_3^-

FIGURE 7-5 ■ Intracellular mechanisms for the movement of ions in acinar and ductule cells of the salivary glands.

exchangers that result in the electroneutral uptake of NaCl. The Na^+ is pumped out of the cell by the ATPase, and Cl^- exits the basolateral surface via an electrogenic Cl^- channel. Some K^+ also enters the cell through a basolateral channel to balance the movement of Cl^-. K^+ enters the lumen in exchange for H^+. An Na^+-H^+ exchanger in the basolateral membrane increases the pH of the cell, driving the Cl^--HCO_3^- exchange at the apical membrane. The tight junctions of the ductule epithelium are relatively impermeable to water when compared with those of the acini. The net result is a decrease in Na^+ and Cl^- concentrations and an increase in K^+ and HCO_3^- concentrations, as well as pH, as the saliva moves down the duct. More ions leave than water (H_2O), and the saliva becomes hypotonic. Aldosterone acts at the luminal membrane to increase the absorption of Na^+ and the secretion of K^+.

Organic Composition

Some organic materials produced and secreted by the salivary glands have been mentioned already in the section describing the functions of saliva. These include the enzymes α-amylase (ptyalin) and lingual lipase, mucus, glycoproteins, lysozymes, and lactoferrin. Another enzyme produced by salivary glands is **kallikrein,** which converts a plasma protein into the potent vasodilator **bradykinin.** Kallikrein is released when the metabolism of the salivary glands increases; it is responsible in part for increased blood flow to the secreting glands. Saliva also contains the blood group substances A, B, AB, and O.

The synthesis of salivary gland enzymes, their storage, and their release are similar to the same processes in the pancreas (detailed in Chapter 9). The protein concentration of saliva is about one tenth the concentration of proteins in the plasma.

REGULATION OF SALIVARY SECRETION

The ANS controls essentially all salivary gland secretion. Antidiuretic hormone (ADH), or vasopressin, and aldosterone modify the composition of saliva by decreasing its Na^+ concentration and increasing its K^+ concentration, but they do not regulate the flow of saliva. The absence of hormonal control of salivation contrasts

with the regulation of the flow of gastric and pancreatic juice and bile. The GI hormones exert major influences on the secretory activity of the stomach, pancreas, and liver. Control of the salivary glands is also unusual in that both the parasympathetic and sympathetic branches stimulate secretion. The parasympathetic system, however, exerts a much greater influence.

Stimulation of the parasympathetic nerves to the salivary glands begins and maintains salivary secretion. Increased secretion results from the activation of transport processes in both acinar and duct cells. Secretion is enhanced by the contraction of the myoepithelial cells that are innervated by the parasympathetic nerves. Parasympathetic fibers also innervate the surrounding blood vessels, stimulating vasodilation and increasing blood flow to the secreting cells. Increased cellular activity in response to parasympathetic stimulation results in increased consumption of glucose and oxygen and the production of vasodilator metabolites. In addition, kallikrein is released, resulting in the production of the vasodilator bradykinin. Increased cellular activity eventually results in growth of the salivary glands. Section of the parasympathetic nerves to the salivary glands causes the glands to atrophy. (These processes are outlined in Figure 7-6.)

Sympathetic activation also stimulates secretion, myoepithelial cell contraction, metabolism, and growth of the salivary glands, although these effects are less pronounced and of shorter duration than those produced by the parasympathetics. Stimulation via the sympathetic nerves produces a biphasic change in blood flow to the salivary glands. The earliest response is a decrease caused by activation of α-adrenergic receptors and vasoconstriction. However, as vasodilator metabolites are produced, blood flow increases over resting levels. Section of the sympathetic fibers to the salivary glands, unlike section of the parasympathetic fibers, has little effect. (The effects of sympathetic stimulation also are summarized in Figure 7-6.)

Salivary glands contain receptors to many mediators, but the most important functionally are the muscarinic cholinergic and β-adrenergic receptors. The parasympathetic mediator is acetylcholine (ACh), which acts on muscarinic receptors, resulting in the formation of inositol triphosphate (IP_3) and the subsequent release of Ca^{++} from intercellular stores. Ca^{++} also may enter the cell from outside. Other agents that

FIGURE 7-6 ■ Summary of the regulation of salivary gland function. ACh, acetylcholine; cAMP, cyclic adenosine monophosphate; CN, cranial nerve; IP$_3$, inositol triphosphate; Norepi, norepinephrine.

are released from neurons in salivary glands and that release Ca^{++} include vasoactive intestinal peptide (VIP) and substance P. The primary sympathetic mediator is norepinephrine, which binds to β-adrenergic receptors, resulting in the formation of cyclic adenosine monophosphate (cAMP). Formation of these second messengers results in protein phosphorylation and enzyme activation that ultimately leads to the stimulation of the salivary glands. In general, agonists that release Ca^{++} have a greater effect on the volume of acinar cell secretion, while those elevating cAMP lead to a greater increase in enzyme and mucus content.

The dual autonomic regulation of the salivary glands is unusual in that the parasympathetic and sympathetic systems both stimulate secretory, metabolic, trophic, muscular, and circulatory functions in similar directions. Their complementary effects are shown in Figure 7-6.

Ultimately, the central nervous system and its autonomic arms are what respond to external events and either stimulate or inhibit activities of the salivary glands. Common events leading to increased glandular activities include chewing, consuming spicy or sour-tasting foods, and smoking. External events leading to glandular inhibition include sleep, fear, dehydration, and fatigue. Glandular activities sensitive to neural control include secretion, circulation, myoepithelial contraction, cellular metabolism, and even parenchymal growth.

Medical conditions likewise can alter either the amount or the composition of saliva. Besides congenital xerostomia (absence of saliva), there is Sjögren's syndrome, an acquired disease characterized by atrophy of the glands and decreased salivation. The commonly used drugs of the digitalis family cause increased concentrations of calcium and potassium in saliva. In cases of cystic fibrosis, salivary sodium, calcium, and protein are elevated (as are these components in the bronchial secretions, pancreatic juice, and sweat of patients with cystic fibrosis). Salivary sodium concentrations also are elevated in Addison's disease, but they are decreased in Cushing's syndrome, in primary aldosteronism, and during pregnancy. These electrolytic changes in saliva reflect events or diseases that make similar alterations in other bodily secretions. Excessive salivation is observed with tumors of the mouth or esophagus and with Parkinson's disease. In these cases, unusual local, reflexive, and more general neurologic stimuli are responsible.

SUMMARY

1. The functions of saliva include those concerned with digestion, protection, and lubrication.
2. Saliva is noteworthy in that it is produced in large volumes relative to the weight of the glands, is hypotonic, and contains relatively high concentrations of K^+.
3. The primary saliva is produced in end pieces called acini and is then modified as it passes through the ducts.
4. Acinar secretion contains ions and water in concentrations approximately equal to those in plasma.
5. Within the ducts, Na^+ and Cl^- are reabsorbed, and K^+ and HCO_3^- are secreted.
6. Because the ductule epithelium is relatively impermeable to water and ions, the saliva becomes more hypotonic as it moves through the ducts.
7. All regulatory control of salivation is provided by the ANS, and both the parasympathetic and sympathetic branches stimulate secretion and metabolism of the glands.

KEY WORDS AND CONCEPTS

- Lubrication
- Protection
- Digestion
- Mucus
- Lysozyme
- Lactoferrin
- Binding glycoprotein for immunoglobulin A
- α-Amylase
- Ptyalin
- Lingual lipase
- Parotid glands
- Submandibular/sublingual glands
- Salivon
- Acinus
- Myoepithelial cells
- Intercalated duct
- Striated duct
- Unique properties
- Kallikrein
- Bradykinin

REFERENCES

Cook DI, van Lennep EW, Roberts M, et al: Secretion by the major salivary glands. In Johnson LR (ed): Physiology of the Gastrointestinal Tract, 3rd ed. New York, Raven Press, 1994.

Melvin JE, Culp DJ: Salivary glands, physiology. In Johnson LR (ed): Encyclopedia of Gastroenterology, vol 3. San Diego, Academic Press, 2004, pp 318-325.

8

GASTRIC SECRETION

LEONARD R. JOHNSON

Four constituents of gastric juice—**intrinsic factor, hydrogen ion, pepsin,** and **mucus**—have physiologic functions. They are secreted by the various cells present within the gastric mucosa. The only indispensable ingredient in gastric juice is intrinsic factor, required for the absorption of vitamin B_{12} by the ileal mucosa. Acid is necessary for the conversion of inactive pepsinogen to the enzyme pepsin. Acid and pepsin begin the digestion of protein, but in their absence pancreatic enzymes hydrolyze all ingested protein, so no nitrogen is wasted in the stools. Acid also kills a large number of bacteria that enter the stomach, thereby reducing the number of organisms reaching the intestine. In cases of severely reduced or absent acid secretion, the incidence of intestinal infections is greater. Mucus lines the wall of the stomach, protecting it from damage. It acts primarily as a lubricant, protecting the mucosa from physical injury. Together with HCO_3^-, mucus neutralizes acid and maintains the surface of the mucosa at a pH near neutrality. This is part of the **gastric mucosal barrier** that protects the stomach from acid and pepsin digestion.

Gastric juice and many of its functions originally were described by a young army surgeon, William Beaumont, stationed at a fort on Mackinac Island in northern Michigan. Beaumont was called to treat a French Canadian, Alexis St. Martin, who had been accidentally shot in the side at close range with a shotgun. St. Martin unexpectedly survived but was left with a permanent opening into his stomach from the outside (gastric fistula). The accident occurred in 1822, and during the ensuing 3 years Beaumont nursed St. Martin back to health. Beaumont retained St. Martin "for the purpose of making physiological experiments," which were begun in 1825. Beaumont's observations and conclusions, many of which remain unchanged today, include the description of the juice itself and its digestive and bacteriostatic functions, the identification of the acid as hydrochloric, the realization that mucus was a separate secretion, the realization that mental disturbances affected gastric function, a direct study of gastric motility, and a thorough study of the ability of gastric juices to digest various foodstuffs.

FUNCTIONAL ANATOMY

Functionally, the gastric mucosa is divided into the **oxyntic gland area** and the **pyloric gland area** (Figure 8-1). The oxyntic gland mucosa secretes acid and is located in the proximal 80% of the stomach. It includes the body and the fundus. The distal 20% of the gastric mucosa, referred to as the *pyloric gland mucosa*, synthesizes and releases the hormone gastrin. This area of the stomach often is designated the **antrum.**

The gastric mucosa is composed of pits and glands (Figure 8-2). The pits and surface itself are lined with mucous or surface epithelial cells. At the base of the pits are the openings of the glands, which project into the mucosa toward the outside or serosa. The oxyntic glands contain the acid-producing **parietal cells** and the **peptic** or **chief cells,** which secrete the enzyme

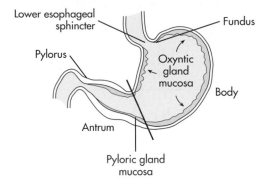

FIGURE 8-1 ■ Areas of the stomach.

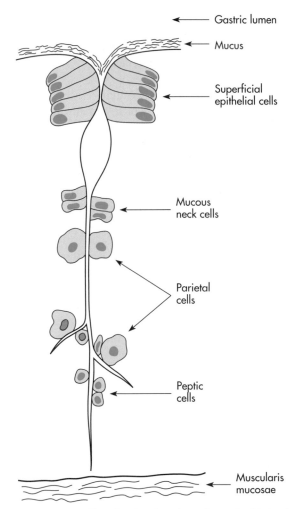

FIGURE 8-2 ■ Oxyntic gland and surface pit. Note the positions of the various cell types.

precursor **pepsinogen.** Pyloric glands contain the gastrin-producing G cells and mucous cells, which also produce pepsinogen. Mucous neck cells are present where the glands open into the pits. Each gland contains a stem cell in this region. These cells divide; one daughter cell remains anchored as the stem cell, and the other divides several times. The resulting new cells migrate both to the surface, where they differentiate into mucous cells, and down into the glands, where they become parietal cells in the oxyntic gland area. Endocrine cells such as the G cells also differentiate from stem cells. Peptic cells are capable of mitosis, but there is evidence that they also can arise from stem cells during the repair of damage to the mucosa. Cells of the surface and pits are replaced much more rapidly than are those of the glands.

The parietal cells secrete hydrochloric acid and, in humans, intrinsic factor. In some species the chief cells also secrete intrinsic factor. The normal human stomach contains approximately 1 billion parietal cells, which produce acid at a concentration of 150 to 160 mEq/L. The number of parietal cells determines the maximal secretory rate and accounts for interindividual variability. The human stomach secretes 1 to 2 L of gastric juice per day. Because the pH of the final juice at high rates of secretion may be less than 1 and that of the blood is 7.4, the parietal cells must expend a large amount of energy to concentrate hydrogen ions. The energy for the production of this more than a million-fold concentration gradient comes from adenosine triphosphate (ATP), produced by the numerous mitochondria located within the cell (Figure 8-3).

During the resting state, the cytoplasm of the parietal cells is dominated by numerous **tubulovesicles.** There is also an **intracellular canaliculus** that is continuous with the lumen of the oxyntic gland. After stimulation of acid secretion, the tubulovesicles become microvilli and project into the canaliculus, which has become greatly expanded to occupy much of the cell. **Carbonic anhydrase** and **H^+,K^+-adenosine triphosphatase** (H^+,K^+-ATPase), enzymes necessary for the production and secretion of acid, are localized in the microvilli. The activities of these enzymes increase during acid secretion. Acid secretion begins within 10 minutes of administering a stimulant. This lag time probably is expended in the morphologic conversion and enzyme activations described previously.

FIGURE 8-3 ■ Parietal cell. **A,** Electron photomicrograph.

Continued

The surface epithelial mucous cells are recognized primarily by the large number of mucous granules at their apical surfaces. During secretion, the membranes of the granules fuse with the cell membrane, expelling mucus.

Peptic cells contain a highly developed endoplasmic reticulum for the synthesis of pepsinogen. The proenzyme is packaged into zymogen granules by the numerous Golgi structures within the cytoplasm. The zymogen granules migrate to the apical surface, where, during secretion, they empty their contents into the lumen by exocytosis. This entire procedure of enzyme synthesis, packaging, and secretion is discussed in greater detail in Chapter 9.

Endocrine cells of the gut also contain numerous granules. Unlike in the peptic and mucous cells, however, these hormone-containing granules are located at the base of the cell. The hormones are secreted into the intercellular space, from which they diffuse into the capillaries. The endocrine cells have numerous microvilli extending from their apical surface into the lumen. Presumably the microvilli contain receptors that sample the luminal contents and trigger hormone secretion in response to the appropriate stimuli.

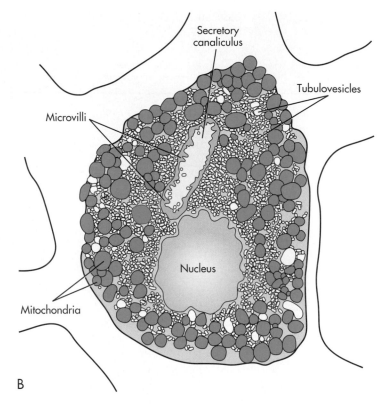

FIGURE 8-3 cont'd ■ **B,** Schematic. *(A, Courtesy of Dr. Bruce MacKay.)*

SECRETION OF ACID

The transport processes involved in the secretion of hydrochloric acid are shown in Figure 8-4. The exact biochemical steps for the production of H^+ are not known, but the reaction can be summarized as follows:

$$HOH \rightarrow OH^- + H^+ \tag{1}$$

$$OH^- + CO_2 \xrightarrow{\text{CA}} HCO_3^- \tag{2}$$

H^+ is pumped actively into the lumen and HCO_3^- diffuses into the blood, giving gastric venous blood a higher pH than that of arterial blood when the stomach is secreting. Step 2 is catalyzed by carbonic anhydrase (CA). Inhibition of this enzyme decreases the rate but does not prevent acid secretion. Metabolism produces much of the CO_2 used to neutralize OH^-, but at high secretory rates, CO_2 from the blood also is required. The active transport of H^+ across the mucosal membrane

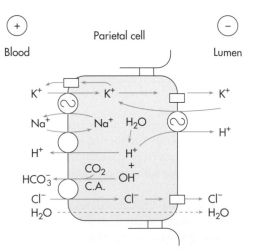

FIGURE 8-4 ■ Transport processes in the gastric mucosa accounting for the presence of the various ions in gastric juice and for the negative transmembrane potential. C.A., carbonic anhydrase.

is catalyzed by H$^+$,K$^+$ ATPase, and H$^+$ is pumped into the lumen in exchange for K$^+$. Within the cell, K$^+$ is accumulated by the Na$^+$,K$^+$-ATPase in the basolateral membrane. Accumulated K$^+$ moves down its electrochemical gradient, leaking across both membranes. Luminal K$^+$ is therefore recycled by the H$^+$,K$^+$-ATPase. Cl$^-$ enters the cell across the basolateral membrane in exchange for HCO$_3^-$. The pumping of H$^+$ out of the cell allows OH$^-$ to accumulate and form HCO$_3^-$ from CO$_2$, a step catalyzed by carbonic anhydrase. The HCO$_3^-$ entering the blood causes the blood's pH to increase, so the gastric venous blood from the actively secreting stomach has a higher pH than arterial blood. The production of OH$^-$ is facilitated by the low intracellular Na$^+$ concentration established by the Na$^+$,K$^+$-ATPase. Some Na$^+$ moves down its gradient back into the cell in exchange for H$^+$, further increasing OH$^-$ production. This in turn increases HCO$_3^-$ production, enhancing the driving force for the entry of Cl$^-$ and its uphill movement from the blood into the lumen. Thus, the movement of Cl$^-$ from blood to lumen against both electrical and chemical gradients is the result of excess OH$^-$ in the cell after the H$^+$ has been pumped out.

The H$^+$,K$^+$-ATPase catalyzes the pumping of H$^+$ out of the cytoplasm into the secretory canaliculus in exchange for K$^+$. The exchange of H$^+$ for K$^+$ has a 1:1 stoichiometry and is therefore electrically neutral. In the resting cell, the H$^+$,K$^+$-ATPase is found in the membranes of the tubulovesicles. Following a secretory stimulus, the tubulovesicles fuse with the canaliculus, greatly increasing the surface area of the secretory membrane and the number of "pumps" in it. When acid secretion ends, the tubulovesicles re-form and the canaliculus shrinks. There is some controversy over whether the tubulovesicles are separate structures or whether they are collapsed canalicular membrane. Most evidence, however, suggests they are separate structures that fuse with the canaliculus and undergo recycling following secretion. H$^+$,K$^+$-ATPase, like Na$^+$, K$^+$-ATPase, with which it has a 60% amino acid homology, is a member of the P-type ion-transporting ATPases, which also include the Ca^{++}-ATPase. Inhibition of the H$^+$,K$^+$-ATPase totally blocks gastric acid secretion. Drugs such as omeprazole, a substituted benzimidazole, are accumulated in acid spaces and are activated at low pH. They then bind irreversibly to sulfhydryl groups of the H$^+$,K$^+$-ATPase, inactivating it. These pump inhibitors are the most potent of the different types of acid secretory inhibitors and are effective agents in the treatment of peptic ulcer, even those caused by a gastrinoma (Zollinger-Ellison syndrome).

ORIGIN OF THE ELECTRICAL POTENTIAL DIFFERENCE

The potential difference across the resting oxyntic gland mucosa is −70 to −80 millivolts (mV) lumen negative with respect to the blood. This charge separation is primarily caused by the secretion of Cl$^-$ (see the previous section) against its electrochemical gradient. This is accomplished by both surface epithelial cells and parietal cells. Following the stimulation of acid secretion, the potential difference decreases to −30 or −40 mV because the positively charged H$^+$ moves in the same direction as Cl$^-$. H$^+$, therefore, is actually secreted down its electrical gradient, facilitating its transport against a several-million-fold concentration gradient.

To produce an electrical gradient and a million-fold concentration gradient of H$^+$, there must be minimal leakage of ions and acid back into the mucosa. The ability of the stomach to prevent leakage is attributed to the so-called gastric mucosal barrier. If this barrier is disrupted by aspirin, alcohol, bile, or a number of agents that damage the gastric mucosa, the potential difference decreases as ions leak down their electrochemical gradients. The exact nature of the barrier is unknown; its properties and the consequences of disrupting it are discussed more fully in the section on the pathophysiology of ulcer diseases (later in this chapter). The negative potential difference across the stomach facilitates acid secretion because H$^+$ is secreted down the electrical gradient. The potential difference can be used to position catheters within the digestive tract. With an electrode placed at the catheter tip, the oxyntic gland mucosa can be distinguished readily from the esophagus (potential difference: −15 mV) or the duodenum (potential difference: −5 mV).

ELECTROLYTES OF GASTRIC JUICE

The concentrations of the major electrolytes in gastric juice are variable, but they are usually related to the rate of secretion (Figure 8-5). At low rates the final juice is

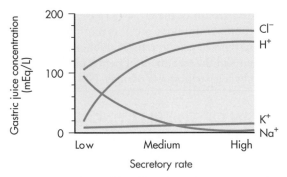

FIGURE 8-5 ■ Relationship of the electrolyte concentrations in gastric juice to the rate of gastric secretion.

essentially a solution of NaCl with small amounts of H^+ and K^+. As the rate increases, the concentration of Na^+ decreases and that of H^+ increases. The concentrations of both Cl^- and K^+ rise slightly as the secretory rate rises. At peak rates, gastric juice is primarily HCl with small amounts of Na^+ and K^+. At all rates of secretion, the concentrations of H^+, K^+, and Cl^- are higher than those in plasma, and the concentration of Na^+ is lower than that in plasma. Thus, gastric juice and plasma—regardless of the secretory rate—are approximately isotonic.

To help understand the changes in ionic concentration, it is convenient to think of gastric juice as a mixture of two separate secretions: a nonparietal component and a parietal component. The nonparietal component is a basal alkaline secretion of constant and low volume. Its primary constituents are Na^+ and Cl^-, and it contains K^+ at about the same concentration as in plasma. In the absence of H^+ secretion, HCO_3^- can be detected in gastric juice. The HCO_3^- is secreted at a concentration of about 30 mEq/L. The nonparietal component is always present, and the parietal component is secreted against this background. As the rate of secretion increases, and because the increase is caused solely by the parietal component, the concentrations of electrolytes in the final juice begin to approach those of pure parietal cell secretion. Pure parietal cell secretion is slightly hyperosmotic and contains 150 to 160 mEq H^+/L and 10 to 20 mEq K^+/L. The only anion present is Cl^-.

This so-called two-component model of gastric secretion is an oversimplification. Parietal secretion is modified somewhat by the exchange of Na^+ for H^+ as the juice moves up the gland into the lumen. Although such changes are minimal, they do participate in determining the final ionic composition of gastric juice.

Knowledge of the composition of gastric juice is required to treat a patient with chronic vomiting or one whose gastric juice is being aspirated and who is being maintained intravenously. Replacement of only NaCl and dextrose will result in hypokalemic metabolic alkalosis, which can be fatal.

STIMULANTS OF ACID SECRETION

Only a few agents directly stimulate the parietal cells to secrete acid. The antral hormone gastrin and the parasympathetic mediator acetylcholine (ACh) are the most important physiologic regulators. ACh stimulates gastrin release in addition to stimulating the parietal cell directly.

Evidence has accumulated that an unknown hormone of intestinal origin also stimulates acid secretion. This substance tentatively has been named *enterooxyntin* to denote both its origin and its action. In humans, circulating amino acids also stimulate the parietal cell and provide some of the stimulation of acid secretion that results from the presence of food in the small intestine.

Histamine, which occurs in many tissues (including the entire gastrointestinal [GI] tract), is a potent stimulator of parietal cell secretion. Histamine release is regulated by gastrin in most mammals, and it in turn stimulates acid secretion in the sense that gastrin and ACh do.

Role of Histamine in Acid Secretion

In 1920 Popielski, a Polish physiologist, discovered that histamine stimulated gastric acid secretion. It was then believed by many that gastrin was actually histamine. The confusion cleared somewhat in 1938 when Komarov demonstrated that there were two separate secretagogues in the gastric mucosa. He showed that trichloroacetic acid precipitated the peptide gastrin from gastric mucosal extracts, leaving histamine in the supernatant. MacIntosh then suggested that histamine was the final common mediator of acid secretion. He proposed that gastrin and ACh released histamine, which in turn stimulated the parietal cells directly and was the only direct stimulant of the parietal cells.

At this point it is important to introduce and define the concept of **potentiation.** Potentiation is said to occur between two stimulants if the response to their simultaneous administration exceeds the sum of the responses when each is administered alone. A number of secretory responses in the GI tract depend on the potentiation of two or more agonists. In the stomach histamine potentiates the effects of gastrin and ACh on the parietal cell. ACh also potentiates the response to gastrin. In this way small amounts of stimuli acting together can often produce a near-maximal secretory response. Potentiation requires the presence of separate receptors on the target cell for each stimulant and, in the case of acid secretion, is incompatible with the final common mediator hypothesis.

The first antihistamines discovered blocked only the histamine H_1 receptor, which mediates actions such as bronchoconstriction and vasodilation. The stimulation of acid secretion by histamine is mediated by the H_2 receptor and is not blocked by conventional antihistamines. The H_2 receptor antagonist, **cimetidine,** effectively inhibits histamine-stimulated acid secretion. Cimetidine, however, has also been found to inhibit the secretory responses to gastrin, ACh, and food. Atropine, a specific antagonist of the muscarinic actions of ACh, decreases the acid responses to gastrin and histamine as well as to ACh. When preparations of isolated parietal cells (which rule out the presence of stimuli other than those directly added) are used, it has been shown that some effects of cimetidine on gastrin- and ACh-stimulated secretion are caused by the inhibition of the part of the secretory response resulting from histamine potentiation. Similarly the inhibition of gastrin- and histamine-stimulated secretion by atropine is caused by removal of the potentiating effects of ACh. Cimetidine is a more effective inhibitor of acid secretion than atropine and has fewer side effects. It is an extremely effective drug for the treatment of duodenal ulcer disease.

Histamine is found in **enterochromaffin-like** (ECL) **cells** within the lamina propria of the gastric glands. The relationships between gastrin, histamine, and ACh are shown in Figure 8-6. Located close to the parietal cells, ECL cells release histamine that acts as a paracrine to stimulate acid secretion. ECL cells have receptors for gastrin and ACh. Gastrin stimulates histamine release and synthesis and the growth of the

FIGURE 8-6 ■ The parietal cell contains receptors for gastrin, acetylcholine (ACh), and histamine. In addition, gastrin and ACh release histamine from the enterochromaffin-like (ECL) cell. AC, adenylate cyclase; cAMP, cyclic adenosine monophosphate; IP_3, inositol triphosphate; PLC, phospholipase C.

ECL cells. ACh also appears to stimulate histamine release. The parietal cell membrane contains receptors for all three agonists. Parietal cells express histamine H_2 receptors, muscarinic M_3 receptors, and gastrin/CCK-2 or B-type receptors. Although gastrin and acetylcholine play central roles in the regulation of acid secretion, in the absence of histamine their effects on the parietal cell are weak.

Gastrin and ACh activate phospholipase C (PLC), which catalyzes the formation of inositol triphosphate (IP_3). IP_3 causes the release of intracellular Ca^{2+}. Histamine activates adenylate cyclase (AC) to form cyclic adenosine monophosphate (cAMP). Ca^{++} and cAMP trigger the events leading to secretion and potentiate each other's effects. Thus the inhibition of acid secretion by histamine H_2 antagonists, such as cimetidine, is due to both removal of potentiative interactions with histamine and inhibition of the stimulation caused by histamine released by gastrin and ACh.

STIMULATION OF ACID SECRETION

The unstimulated human stomach secretes acid at a rate equal to 10% to 15% of that present during maximal stimulation. Basal acid secretion exhibits a diurnal rhythm with higher rates in the evening and lower rates in the morning before awakening. The cause of the diurnal variation is unknown, since plasma gastrin is relatively constant during the interdigestive phase. The stomach emptied of food therefore contains a relatively small volume of gastric juice, and the pH of this fluid is usually less than 2. Thus in the absence of food the gastric mucosa is acidified.

The stimulation of gastric secretion is conveniently divided into three phases based on the location of the receptors initiating the secretory responses. It is important to realize that this division is artificial; shortly after the start of a meal, stimulation is initiated from all three areas at the same time.

Cephalic Phase

Chemoreceptors and mechanoreceptors located in the tongue and the buccal and nasal cavities are stimulated by tasting, smelling, chewing, and swallowing food. The afferent nerve impulses are relayed through the vagal nucleus and vagal efferent fibers to the stomach. Even the thought of an appetizing meal stimulates gastric secretion. The secretory response to cephalic stimulation depends greatly on the nature of the meal. The greatest response occurs to an appetizing self-selected meal. A bland meal produces a much smaller response. The efferent pathway for the cephalic phase is the vagus nerve. The entire response is blocked by vagotomy.

The cephalic phase is best studied by the procedure known as *sham feeding*. A dog is prepared with esophageal and gastric fistulas. When the esophageal fistula is open, swallowed food falls to the exterior without entering the stomach. Gastric secretion is collected from the gastric fistula, and its volume and acid content are measured. Stimulation during the cephalic phase represents about 30% of the total response to a meal. The cephalic phase also can be studied using a variety of drugs. Hypoglycemia introduced by tolbutamide or insulin, or interference with glucose metabolism by glucose analogues such as 3-methylglucose or 2-deoxyglucose, activates hypothalamic centers that stimulate secretion via the vagus nerve.

The vagus acts directly on the parietal cells to stimulate acid secretion. It also acts on the antral gastrin cells (G cells) to stimulate gastrin release. The mediator at the parietal cells is ACh. The mediator at the gastrin cell appears to be **gastrin-releasing peptide** (GRP) or **bombesin.** Within the antrum, postganglionic vagal neurons release both stimulatory and inhibitory neurotransmitters. All of these have not been identified, and the overall response is the result of a complex process. The direct effect on the parietal cell is the more important in humans, for selective vagotomy of the parietal cell–containing area of the stomach abolishes the response to sham feeding, whereas antrectomy only moderately reduces it. The mechanisms involved in the cephalic phase are illustrated in Figure 8-7.

Gastric Phase

Acid secretion during the gastric phase accounts for at least 50% of the response to a meal. When swallowed food first enters the stomach and mixes with the small volume of juice normally present, buffers

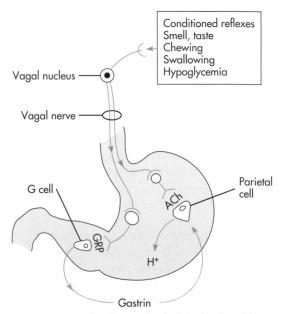

FIGURE 8-7 ■ Mechanisms stimulating gastric acid secretion during the cephalic phase. ACh, acetylcholine; G cell, gastrin-producing cell; GRP, gastrin-releasing peptide.

(primarily protein) contained in the food neutralize the acid. The pH of the gastric contents may rise to 6 or above. Because gastrin release is inhibited when the antral pH drops below 3 and is prevented totally when the pH is less than 2, essentially no gastrin is released from a stomach that is void of food. The rise in pH permits vagal stimulation from the cephalic phase to initiate, and stimuli from the gastric phase to maintain, gastrin release. It is important to realize that increasing the pH of the gastric contents is not, in itself, a stimulus for gastrin release but merely allows other stimuli to be effective.

Distention of the stomach and bathing the gastric mucosa with certain chemicals, primarily amino acids and peptides, are the effective stimuli of the gastric phase. Distention activates mechanoreceptors in the mucosa of both the oxyntic and the pyloric gland areas. It also may activate long extramural reflexes or local short intramural reflexes. All distention reflexes are mediated cholinergically and can be blocked by atropine.

Long reflexes also are called **vagovagal reflexes,** meaning that both afferent impulses and efferent impulses are carried by neurons in the vagus nerve. Mucosal distention receptors send signals by vagal afferents to the vagal nucleus. Efferent signals are sent back to G cells and parietal cells by the vagal efferents.

Short or local reflexes are mediated by neurons that are contained entirely within the wall of the stomach. These may be single-neuron reflexes, or they may involve intermediary neurons. There are two local distention reflexes. Both of these are regional reflexes, meaning that the receptor and effector are located in the same area of the stomach. Distention of a vagally innervated pyloric (antrum) pouch stimulates gastrin release. The effect is decreased, but not abolished, by vagotomy, meaning that the gastrin response is mediated by both vagovagal reflexes and local reflexes. This local reflex is called a *pyloropyloric reflex.*

Distention of an antral pouch with pH 1 hydrochloric acid stimulates acid secretion from the oxyntic gland area. Because gastrin release does not take place when the pH is below 2, the increase in acid output must be mediated by a neural reflex. As the discerning reader will have surmised, this vagovagal reflex is known as a *pyloro-oxyntic reflex.* Distention reflexes, which are much more effective stimulants of the parietal cell than they are of the G cell, are illustrated diagrammatically in Figure 8-8.

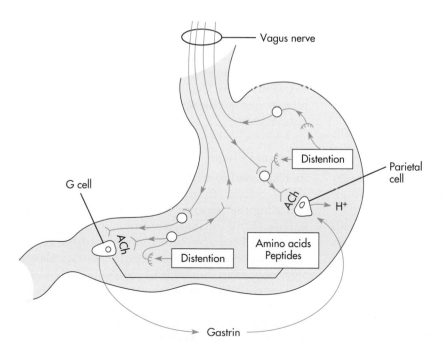

FIGURE 8-8 ■ Mechanisms stimulating gastric acid secretion during the gastric phase. ACh, acetylcholine; G cell, gastrin-producing cell.

Peptides and amino acids stimulate gastrin release from the G cells. The most potent of these releasers are the aromatic amino acids. This effect is not blocked by vagotomy. Only part of it appears to be blocked by atropine, indicating that protein digestion products contain chemicals capable of directly stimulating the G cell to release gastrin. Acidification of the antral mucosa below pH 3 inhibits gastrin release in response to digested protein. A few other commonly ingested substances are also capable of stimulating acid secretion. Caffeine stimulates the parietal cells directly. Calcium, either in the gastric lumen or as elevated serum concentrations, stimulates gastrin release and acid secretion. Considerable debate exists about the effects of alcohol on gastric secretion. Alcohol has been shown to stimulate gastrin release and acid secretion in some species; however, these effects do not seem appear to occur in humans.

Release of Gastrin

Considerable evidence has accumulated favoring a mechanism similar to that in Figure 8-9 to explain the regulation of gastrin release. GRP acts on the G cell to stimulate gastrin release, and **somatostatin** acts on the G cell to inhibit release. GRP is a neurocrine released by vagal stimulation. This explains why atropine does not block vagally mediated gastrin release. Somatostatin acts as a paracrine, and its release is inhibited by vagal stimulation. In the isolated, perfused rat stomach, vagal stimulation increases GRP release and decreases somatostatin release into the perfusate. Thus it appears that vagal activation stimulates gastrin by releasing GRP and inhibiting the release of somatostatin. Some recent evidence from studies involving a GRP receptor antagonist brings into question the role of GRP. These data indicate that although GRP is involved in vagally mediated acid secretion, it may not be responsible for the release of gastrin.

Acid in the lumen of the stomach is believed to act directly on the somatostatin cell to stimulate the release of somatostatin, thereby preventing gastrin release. Protein digestion products—peptides, amino acids, and amines—may act directly on the G cell (or be absorbed by the G cell) to stimulate gastrin release. These substances most likely bind to receptors located on the apical membrane of the G cells, which are in contact with the gastric lumen.

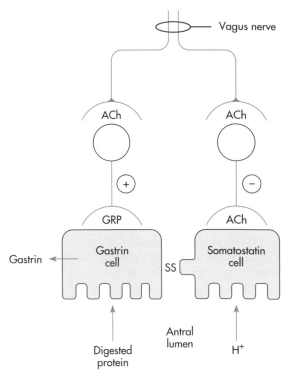

FIGURE 8-9 ■ Mechanism for the regulation of gastrin release. ACh, acetylcholine; GRP, gastrin-releasing peptide; SS, somatostatin.

There are data indicating that atropine can block some gastrin release stimulated by protein digestion products. This is evidence that luminal receptors may be activated, resulting in a cholinergic reflex that leads to gastrin release. There is also evidence that this reflex may operate by releasing GRP and inhibiting somatostatin release.

Intestinal Phase

Protein digestion products in the duodenum stimulate acid secretion from denervated gastric mucosa, indicating the presence of a hormonal mechanism. In humans, the proximal duodenum is rich in gastrin, which has been shown to contribute to the serum gastrin response to a meal. In dogs, liver extract releases a hormone from the duodenal mucosa that stimulates acid secretion without increasing serum gastrin levels. This hormone tentatively has been named *enterooxyntin*. Its significance in humans is unknown.

Intravenous infusion of amino acids has recently been shown to stimulate acid secretion. Therefore a good portion of the stimulation attributed to the intestinal phase may be caused by absorbed amino acids. Intestinal stimuli result in only about 5% of the acid response to a meal. The gastric phase is responsible for most acid secretion.

Figure 8-10 summarizes the mechanisms and final stimulants acting in all three phases.

INHIBITION OF ACID SECRETION

When food first enters the stomach, its buffers neutralize the small volume of gastric acid present during the interdigestive phase. As the pH of the antral mucosa rises above 3, gastrin is released by the stimuli of the cephalic and gastric phases. One hour after the meal, the rate of gastric secretion is maximal, the buffering capacity of the meal is saturated, a significant portion of the meal has emptied from the stomach, and the acid concentration of the gastric contents increases. As the pH falls, gastrin release is inhibited, removing a

significant factor for the stimulation of gastric acid secretion. This passive negative feedback mechanism is extremely important in the regulation of acid secretion. In addition, somatostatin released by the drop in intragastric pH also directly inhibits the parietal cells.

Evidence exists for several hormonal mechanisms for the active inhibition of gastric acid secretion. These hormones are released from duodenal mucosa by acid, fatty acids, or hyperosmotic solutions and collectively are termed **enterogastrones.** They often inhibit gastric emptying as well as acid secretion. Teleologically these mechanisms ensure that the gastric contents are delivered to the small bowel at a rate that does not exceed the capacity for digestion and absorption. They also prevent damage to the duodenal mucosa that can result from acidic and hyperosmotic solutions.

Gastric inhibitory peptide (GIP) is released by fatty acids and acts at the parietal cell to inhibit acid secretion. **Secretin** may also be classified as an enterogastrone because it too inhibits gastric acid

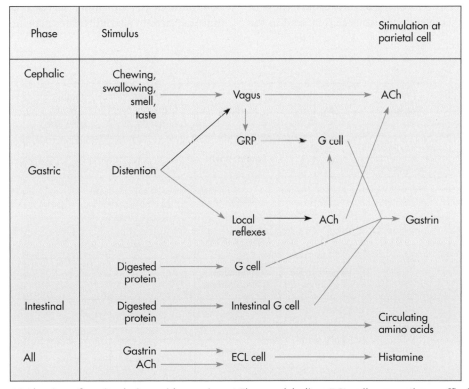

FIGURE 8-10 ■ Mechanisms for stimulating acid secretion. ACh, acetylcholine; ECL cell, enterochromaffin-like cell; GRP, gastrin-releasing peptide.

secretion. The importance and physiologic significance of these effects in humans have not been determined. **Cholecystokinin** (CCK) is a physiologically significant inhibitor of gastric emptying. Hyperosmotic solutions release an as yet unidentified enterogastrone. Strong evidence also exists that acid initiates a nervous reflex from receptors in the duodenal mucosa that suppresses acid secretion. These mechanisms are summarized in Figure 8-11.

PEPSIN

Pepsinogen has a molecular weight of 42,500 and is split to form the active enzyme pepsin, which has a molecular weight of 35,000. Pepsinogen is converted to pepsin in the gastric juice when the pH drops below 5. Pepsin itself can catalyze the formation of additional pepsin from pepsinogen. Pepsin begins the digestion of protein by splitting interior peptide linkages (see Chapter 11).

Pepsinogens belong to two main groups: I and II. The pepsinogens in the first group are secreted by peptic and mucous cells of the oxyntic glands; those in the second are secreted by mucous cells present in the pyloric gland area and duodenum, as well as in the oxyntic gland area. Pepsinogens appear in the blood, and there is considerable evidence that their levels may be correlated with duodenal ulcer formation. This is discussed in connection with peptic ulcer disease (later in this chapter).

The strongest stimulant of pepsinogen secretion is ACh. Thus vagal activation during both the cephalic and the gastric phase results in a significant proportion of the total pepsinogen secreted. Hydrogen ion plays an important role in several areas of pepsin physiology. First, acid is necessary to convert pepsinogen to the active enzyme pepsin. At pH 2 this conversion is almost instantaneous. Second, acid triggers a local cholinergic reflex that stimulates the chief cells to secrete. This mechanism is atropine sensitive and may account in part for the strong correlation between acid and pepsin outputs. Third, the acid-sensitive reflex greatly enhances the effects of other stimuli on the peptic cell. This mechanism ensures that large amounts of pepsinogen are not secreted unless sufficient acid for conversion to pepsin is present. Fourth, acid releases the hormone secretin from duodenal mucosa. Secretin also stimulates pepsinogen secretion,

Region	Stimulus	Mediator	Inhibit gastrin release	Inhibit acid secretion
Oxyntic glands	Acid (pH <3.0)	Somatostatin		+
Antrum			+	
Duodenum	Acid	Secretin	+	+
		Nervous reflex		+
	Hyperosmotic solutions	Unidentified enterogastrone		+
Duodenum and jejunum	Fatty acids	GIP	+	+
		Unidentified enterogastrone		+

FIGURE 8-11 ■ Mechanisms for inhibiting acid secretion. GIP, gastric inhibitory peptide.

although it is questionable whether enough secretin is present to do so under normal conditions.

The hormone gastrin is usually listed as a pepsigogue. Infusion of gastrin increases pepsin secretion. In dogs, the entire response can be accounted for by the stimulation of acid secretion by gastrin and the subsequent activation of the acid-sensitive reflex mechanism for pepsinogen secretion. In humans, gastrin may be a weak pepsigogue in its own right. The mechanisms regulating pepsinogen secretion are summarized in Figure 8-12.

Pepsin plays an important role in the ulceration of the stomach and duodenum—hence the term "peptic ulcer." In the absence of pepsin, gastric acid does not produce an ulcer. Thus, one of the benefits of the inhibition of acid secretion or neutralization of gastric acid during ulcer therapy may be the elimination of pepsin.

MUCUS

Vagal nerve stimulation and ACh increase soluble mucus secretion from the mucous neck cells. Soluble mucus consists of mucoproteins and mixes with the gastric chyme lubricating it.

Surface mucous cells secrete visible or insoluble mucus in response to chemical stimulants (such as ethanol) and in response to physical contact and friction with roughage in the diet. Visible mucus is secreted as a gel that entraps the alkaline component of the surface cell secretion. It is present during the interdigestive phase and protects the mucosa with an alkaline layer of lubricant. A portion of this coating is made up of mucus-containing surface cells that have been shed and trapped in the layer of mucus. During the response to a meal, insoluble mucus protects the mucosa from physical and chemical damage. It neutralizes a certain amount of acid and prevents pepsin from coming into contact with the mucosa. On contact with acid, insoluble mucus precipitates into clumps and passes into the duodenum with the chyme.

INTRINSIC FACTOR

Intrinsic factor is a mucoprotein with a molecular weight of 55,000 that is secreted by the parietal cells. It combines with vitamin B_{12} in the stomach, forming a complex that is necessary for the absorption of this vitamin by the ileal mucosa. Failure to secrete intrinsic

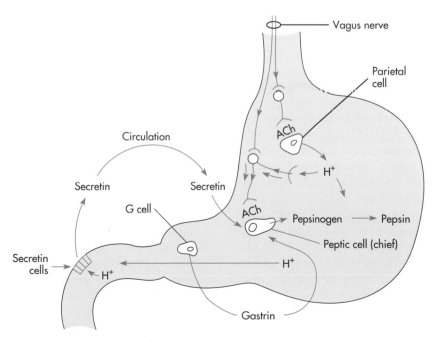

FIGURE 8-12 ■ Summary of mechanisms for stimulating pepsinogen secretion and activation to pepsin. ACh, acetylcholine.

factor is associated with achlorhydria and the absence of parietal cells, which results in vitamin B_{12} deficiency or pernicious anemia. The development of this disease is poorly understood, for the liver stores enough vitamin B_{12} to last several years. The disease therefore is not recognized until long after the changes have taken place in the gastric mucosa.

GROWTH OF THE MUCOSA

The growth of the GI mucosa is influenced by non-GI hormones and factors associated with the ingestion and digestion of a meal, such as GI hormones, nervous stimulation, secretions, and trophic substances present in the diet. Hypophysectomy results in atrophy of the digestive tract mucosa and the pancreas. The effects of hypophysectomy on growth can be prevented by administration of growth hormone. When administered to hypophysectomized rats, gastrin prevents atrophy of the GI mucosa and exocrine pancreas but does not affect the growth of other tissues. There is interesting evidence that adrenocortical steroids may trigger early postnatal development of the GI tract.

Gastrin is an important and necessary regulator of the growth of the oxyntic gland mucosa. It also stimulates growth of the intestinal and colonic mucosa and the exocrine pancreas. In humans, antrectomy causes atrophy of the remaining gastric mucosa; in rats, it causes atrophy of all GI mucosa (except that of the antrum and esophagus) and the exocrine pancreas. These changes are prevented by administration of exogenous gastrin. Hypergastrinemia results primarily in an increase in parietal and ECL cells. Gastrin is a potent stimulator of ECL cell proliferation, and prolonged hypergastrinemia leads to ECL cell hyperplasia.

Disruption of gastrin gene expression in mice inhibits parietal cell maturation and decreases their number. On the other hand, overexpression of the gene results in increased proliferation of the gastric epithelium, increased number of parietal cells, and increased acid secretion. Partial resection of the small intestine for tumor removal or for a variety of other reasons (such as treatment of morbid obesity) results in adaptation of the remaining mucosa. The mucosa of the entire digestive tract undergoes hyperplasia, which increases its ability to digest and transport nutrients or, in the case of the stomach, to secrete acid.

Resection increases gastrin levels but not sufficiently to account for the adaptive changes. There is evidence that increased exposure of the mucosa to luminal contents plays an important role. After removal of proximal intestine, the distal intact mucosa is exposed to an increased load of pancreatic juice, bile, and nutrients. Investigators have hypothesized that bile and pancreatic juice contain growth factors that stimulate the adaptive response. The growth factors have not been isolated and tested. Increased uptake of nutrients by the distal mucosa has also been hypothesized to result in growth. Effects of specific nutrients have not been proved, and there is disagreement whether growth is caused by an increased workload or an increase in the available supply of calories. Good evidence exists that a hormone different from gastrin also is involved in the adaptive response. This may be one of the glucagon-like peptides released from the distal small intestine.

The diet also contains polyamines that are required for growth. Trophic agents like gastrin stimulate polyamine synthesis in the proliferative cells. Thus increased luminal polyamines from the diet, coupled with synthesis stimulated by trophic hormones, may explain the regulation of mucosal growth triggered by changes in the diet.

PATHOPHYSIOLOGY

Gastric and duodenal ulcers are lumped together under the heading of peptic ulcer disease. Although formation of both types of ulcer requires acid and pepsin, their etiologies are basically different. Quite simply, an ulcer forms when damage from acid and pepsin overcomes the ability of the mucosa to protect itself and replace damaged cells. In the case of gastric ulcer the defect is more often in the ability of the mucosa to withstand injury. In the case of duodenal ulcer there is good evidence that the mucosa is exposed to increased amounts of acid and pepsin. This analysis is an oversimplification, for both factors are no doubt important in all cases of ulcer.

Representative acid secretory rates for normal individuals and patients with GI disorders are shown in Table 8-1. Maximal acid secretory output sometimes is measured but, in itself, is of little value in diagnosing ulcer disease. Normal subjects secrete approximately 25 mEq H^+/hour, in response to maximal injection of

TABLE 8-1

Comparison of Acid Output Values from the Human Stomach*

CONDITION	REPRESENTATIVE RANGES	
	Basal Acid Output (mEq/hr)	Maximal Acid Output (mEq/hr)
Normal	1 to 5	6 to 40
Gastric ulcer	0 to 3	1 to 20
Pernicious anemia	0	0 to 10
Duodenal ulcer	2 to 10	15 to 60
Zollinger-Ellison syndrome (gastrinoma)	10 to 30	30 to 80

*Basal acid output occurs at rest, and maximal acid output occurs during stimulation with histamine. The value is determined by multiplying the hourly volume of gastric juice aspirated times the hydrogen ion concentration of the juice.

histamine, betazole, or gastrin. The mean output of patients with duodenal ulcer disease is approximately 40 mEq H+/hour, but the degree of overlap between individuals is so great as to render the determination useless in diagnosis. The highest rates of acid secretion are seen in cases of gastrinoma (Zollinger-Ellison syndrome), but again individual overlap makes it impossible to differentiate between this condition and duodenal ulcer on the basis of secretory data alone. Lower than normal secretory rates are found in cases of gastric ulcer, and still lower secretory rates are found in patients with gastric carcinoma. Many patients in the latter two groups, however, fall well within the normal range.

Because of the feedback mechanism whereby antral acidification inhibits gastrin release, the general statement can be made that serum gastrin levels are related inversely to acid secretory capacity. Patients with gastric ulcer and carcinoma usually have higher than normal serum gastrin levels. Serum gastrin levels in pernicious anemia actually may approach those seen in gastrinoma. Obviously, gastrinoma patients are an exception to this rule because their hypergastrinemia is derived not from the antrum but from a tumor not subject to inhibition by gastric acid. Except for the special tests mentioned in Chapter 1, serum gastrin levels cannot be used to differentiate various secretory abnormalities.

The decreased rate of acid secretion experienced with gastric ulcer is caused in part by the failure to recover acid that has been secreted and then has leaked back across the damaged gastric mucosa. (The concept of the gastric mucosal barrier is illustrated in Figure 8-13.) The normal gastric mucosa is relatively impermeable to H+. If the gastric mucosal barrier is weakened or damaged, H+ leaks into the mucosa in exchange for Na+. As H+ accumulates in the mucosa, intracellular buffers are saturated, and the intracellular pH decreases, resulting in injury and cell death. Potassium leaks from the damaged cells into the lumen. H+ damages mucosal mast cells. They then release histamine, which exacerbates the condition by acting on the mucosal capillaries. The result is local ischemia,

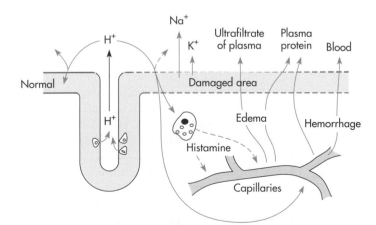

FIGURE 8-13 ■ Events that follow damage to the gastric mucosal barrier.

hypoxia, and vascular stasis. Plasma proteins and pepsin leak into the gastric juice; if damage is severe, bleeding occurs. Common agents that produce mucosal damage of this type are aspirin, ethanol, and bile salts. The mucosal lesions produced by topical damage to the gastric barrier may be forerunners of gastric ulcer.

The exact nature of the barrier is unknown. It is probably physiologic as well as anatomic. Cell membranes and junctional complexes prevent normal back-diffusion of H^+. Diffused H^+ normally is transported actively back into the lumen. Factors that have been speculated to play a role in maintaining mucosal resistance are blood flow, mucus, bicarbonate secretion, cellular renewal, and chemical factors such as gastrin, prostaglandins, and epidermal growth factor. The last three agents have all been shown to decrease the severity and promote the healing of gastric ulcers.

Factors that have been elucidated as important in duodenal ulcer formation pertain to acid and pepsin secretion. Duodenal ulcer patients have on the average 2 billion parietal cells and can secrete about 40 mEq H^+/hour. Comparable measurements for normal individuals are about 50% of this. In addition, the secretion of pepsin is doubled in the duodenal ulcer group, as can be detected by measuring plasma pepsinogen. Although fasting serum gastrin is normal in patients with duodenal ulcer, gastrin response to a meal and sensitivity to gastrin are increased. Increased serum gastrin after a meal is caused in part by the fact that acid suppresses gastrin release less effectively in duodenal ulcer patients than in controls. The increased parietal cell mass may therefore by caused by the trophic effect of gastrin.

Work done during the last several years has established that the major acquired factor in the etiology of both gastric and duodenal ulcer is the bacterium *Helicobacter pylori*. The infection is found in 80% of patients with duodenal ulcer and virtually 100% of patients with gastric ulcers whose ulcers were not caused by chronic use of aspirin or other nonsteroidal anti-inflammatory drugs (NSAIDs). *H. pylori* is a gram-negative bacterium, characterized by a high urease activity, which metabolizes urea into ammonia to neutralize gastric acid. This reaction allows the bacterium to withstand the acid environment of the stomach and to colonize the mucosa. The resulting production of NH_4^+ is believed to be a major cause of cytotoxicity, because NH_4^+ directly damages epithelial cells and increases the permeability of the mucosa (i.e., it "breaks the mucosal barrier"). The bacteria produce numerous other factors, such as cytokines, that also damage cells. All of these probably contribute to gastric ulcer formation.

H. pylori also appears to cause the increased acid secretion associated with duodenal ulcer. A recent study found that, when compared with normal individuals, patients with duodenal ulcer had increased basal acid output, increased GRP-stimulated acid output, increased maximal acid output in response to gastrin, increased ratio of basal acid output to gastrin-stimulated maximal acid output, and increased ratio of GRP-stimulated maximal acid output to gastrin-stimulated maximal acid output. All of these, except the increased maximal acid output in response to gastrin, totally disappeared following eradication of the *H. pylori* infection. The increased acid secretory and serum gastrin responses to GRP appear to be related to a decreased inhibition of gastrin release and parietal cell secretion by somatostatin in *H. pylori*–infected persons. Patterns of *H. pylori*–related gastritis differ in gastric and duodenal ulcer. Gastric ulcers are associated with a diffuse gastritis, whereas duodenal ulcers are associated predominantly with the infection of the antrum. Although all of the mechanisms by which *H. pylori* affects the mucosa have not been elucidated, the information available appears to coincide with the known pathophysiology of both gastric and duodenal ulcer diseases.

Medical treatment of duodenal ulcer disease usually consists of administering antacids to neutralize secreted acid or a histamine H_2 receptor blocker to inhibit secretion. The H^+,K^+-ATPase (H^+ pump) inhibitor omeprazole blocks all acid secretion. It is extremely effective in treating duodenal ulcers, even those caused by gastrinoma. Surgical treatment is based entirely on physiology. The most commonly used operations are vagotomy and/or antrectomy. These procedures result in a 60% to 70% decrease in acid secretion by removing one or both major stimulants of acid secretion and their potentiating interaction. With the advent of the H_2 blockers and omeprazole, ulcers are now rarely treated by surgical intervention. To prevent recurrence, physicians also try to eradicate *H. pylori*. This is best done by giving antibiotics in combination with omeprazole, which increases the susceptibility of the bacteria to antibiotic treatment.

SUMMARY

1. The functions of gastric juice are attributed to acid, pepsin, intrinsic factor, and mucus.

2. Acid is secreted in concentrations as high as 150 mEq/L at high rates of secretion; the acid converts inactive pepsinogen to the active enzyme pepsin, kills bacteria, and solubilizes some food-stuffs.

3. Acid is secreted by the parietal cells, which contain the enzyme H^+,K^+-ATPase on their apical secretory membranes.

4. The concentrations of the electrolytes in gastric juice vary with the rate of secretion.

5. The three major stimulants of acid secretion are the hormone gastrin, the cholinergic neuromediator ACh, and the paracrine histamine, which is released from ECL cells in response to gastrin and ACh.

6. During the cephalic phase of secretion, vagal activation stimulates the parietal cells directly via ACh and releases gastrin from the G cells.

7. During the gastric phase of secretion, distention of the wall of the stomach stimulates the parietal cells and releases gastrin via both mucosal and vagovagal reflexes; protein digestion products stimulate the G cells directly to release gastrin.

8. When the pH of luminal contents drops below 3, somatostatin is released from D cells in the antrum and oxyntic gland area, where it inhibits gastrin release and acid secretion, respectively.

9. Acid secretion is inhibited further when chyme enters the duodenum and triggers the release of inhibitory hormones and initiates inhibitory neural reflexes.

10. Pepsinogen secretion is stimulated by vagal activation and ACh and by acid in the lumen of the stomach.

11. Intrinsic factor, secreted by the parietal cells, is required for the absorption of vitamin B_{12} by a specific carrier mechanism located in the ileum.

KEY WORDS AND CONCEPTS

- Intrinsic factor
- Hydrogen ion
- Pepsin
- Mucus
- Gastric mucosal barrier
- Oxyntic gland area
- Pyloric gland area
- Antrum
- Parietal cells
- Peptic/chief cells
- Pepsinogen
- Tubulovesicles
- Intracellular canaliculus
- Carbonic anhydrase
- H^+,K^+-ATPase
- Histamine
- Potentiation
- Cimetidine
- Enterochromaffin-like cells
- Gastrin-releasing peptide/bombesin
- Vagovagal reflexes
- Somatostatin
- Enterogastrones
- Gastric inhibitory peptide
- Secretin
- Cholecystokinin

REFERENCES

Beaumont W: Experiments and Observations on the Gastric Juice and the Physiology of Digestion. New York, Dover, 1955.

Chan FK, Leung WK: Peptic ulcer disease. Lancet 360:933-940, 2002.

El-Omar EM, Penman ID, Ardill JES, et al: *Helicobacter pylori* infection and abnormalities of acid secretion in patients with duodenal ulcer disease. Gastroenterology 109:681-691, 1995.

Feldman M, Richardson CT: Gastric acid secretion in humans. In Johnson LR (ed): Physiology of the Gastrointestinal Tract. New York, Raven Press, 1981.

Forte JG, Wolosin JM: HCl secretion by the gastric oxyntic cell. In Johnson LR (ed): Physiology of the Gastrointestinal Tract, 2nd ed. New York, Raven Press, 1987.

Hersey SJ: Gastric secretion of pepsinogens. In Johnson LR (ed): Physiology of the Gastrointestinal Tract, 3rd ed. New York, Raven Press, 1994.

Johnson LR, McCormack SA: Regulation of gastrointestinal growth. In Johnson LR (ed): Physiology of the Gastrointestinal Tract, 3rd ed. New York, Raven Press, 1994.

Lindström E, Chen D, Norlen P, et al: Control of gastric acid secretion: The gastrin–ECL cell–parietal cell axis. Comp Biol Physiol Part A Mol Integr Physiol 128:505-514, 2001.

Lloyd KCK, Debas HT: Peripheral regulation of gastric acid secretion. In Johnson LR (ed): Physiology of the Gastrointestinal Tract, 3rd ed. New York, Raven Press, 1994.

Modlin IM, Sachs G: Acid Related Diseases. Milan, Schnetztor-Verlag Gmbh D-Konstanz, 1998.

Sachs G: The gastric H^+,K^+-ATPase: Regulation and structure/function of the acid pump of the stomach. In Johnson LR (ed): Physiology of the Gastrointestinal Tract, 3rd ed. New York, Raven Press, 1994.

Saffouri B, DuVal JW, Makhlouf GM: Stimulation of gastrin secretion in vitro by intraluminal chemicals: Regulation by intramural cholinergic and noncholinergic neurons. Gastroenterology 87:557-561, 1984.

Silen W: Gastric mucosal defense and repair. In Johnson LR (ed): Physiology of the Gastrointestinal Tract, 2nd ed. New York, Raven Press, 1987.

9 PANCREATIC SECRETION

LEONARD R. JOHNSON

P ancreatic exocrine secretion is divided conveniently into an aqueous or bicarbonate component and an enzymatic component. The function of the **aqueous component** is the neutralization of the duodenal contents. As such, it prevents damage to the duodenal mucosa by acid and pepsin and brings the pH of the contents into the optimum range for activity of the pancreatic enzymes. The **enzymatic** or **protein component** is a low-volume secretion containing enzymes for the digestion of all normal constituents of a meal. Unlike the enzymes secreted by the stomach and salivary glands, the pancreatic enzymes are essential to normal digestion and absorption.

FUNCTIONAL ANATOMY

The exocrine pancreas can best be likened to a cluster of grapes, and its functional units resemble the salivons of the salivary glands. Groups of acini form lobules separated by areolar tissue. Each acinus is formed from several pyramidal **acinar cells** oriented with their apices toward the lumen. The lumen of the spherical acinus is drained by a ductule whose epithelium extends into the acinus in the form of centroacinar cells. Ductules join to form intralobular ducts, which in turn drain into interlobular ducts. These join the major pancreatic duct draining the gland.

The acinar cells secrete a small volume of juice rich in protein. Essentially all of the proteins present in pancreatic juice are digestive enzymes. **Ductule cells** and **centroacinar cells** produce a large volume of watery secretion containing Na^+ and HCO_3^- as its major constituents.

Distributed throughout the pancreatic parenchyma are the **islets of Langerhans** or the endocrine pancreas. The islets produce insulin from the β cells and glucagon from the α cells. In addition, the pancreas produces the candidate hormone pancreatic polypeptide and contains large amounts of somatostatin, which may act as a paracrine to inhibit the release of insulin and glucagon.

The efferent nerve supply to the pancreas includes both sympathetics and parasympathetics. Sympathetic postganglionic fibers emanate from the celiac and superior mesenteric plexuses and accompany the arteries to the organ. Parasympathetic preganglionic fibers are distributed by branches of the vagi coursing down the antral-duodenal region. Hence, surgical vagotomy for peptic ulcer disease affects not only the intended target organ, the hypersecreting stomach, but also the pancreas. Recently, more selective operations have been designed to resect only the vagal branches passing to the stomach. Vagal fibers terminate either at acini and islets or at the intrinsic cholinergic nerves of the pancreas. In general, the sympathetic nerves inhibit, and the parasympathetic nerves stimulate, pancreatic exocrine secretion.

MECHANISMS OF FLUID AND ELECTROLYTE SECRETION

The pancreas secretes approximately 1 liter (L) of fluid per day. At all rates of secretion, pancreatic juice is

85

essentially isotonic with extracellular fluid. At low rates the primary ions are Na^+ and Cl^-. At high rates Na^+ and HCO_3^- predominate. Potassium ions are present at all rates of secretion at a concentration equal to their concentration in plasma. The concentrations of Na^+ in pancreatic juice and in plasma also are approximately equal.

The aqueous component is secreted by the ductule and centroacinar cells and may contain 120 to 140 milliequivalents (mEq) of HCO_3^-/L, several times its concentration in plasma. The electropotential difference across the ductule epithelium is 5 to 9 millivolts (mV), lumen negative. Hence HCO_3^- is secreted against both electrical and chemical gradients. This is often considered evidence that HCO_3^- is transported actively across the luminal surface of the cells. Although the exact mechanism involved in pancreatic HCO_3^- secretion is unknown, one current model is shown in Figure 9-1. This model is based on information that shows the following: (1) over 90% of HCO_3^- in pancreatic juice is derived from plasma; (2) the secretion of HCO_3^- occurs against an electrochemical gradient and is an active process; (3) HCO_3^- secretion is blocked by ouabain, meaning that the Na^+,K^+-ATPase is involved; (4) HCO_3^- secretion involves Na^+-H^+ and Cl^--HCO_3^- exchangers and carbonic anhydrase; and (5) HCO_3^- secretion is decreased significantly in the absence of extracellular Cl^-. The initial step in Figure 9-1 is the diffusion of CO_2 into the cell, its hydration by carbonic anhydrase, and its dissociation into H^+ and HCO_3^-. The H^+ is transported across the basolateral membrane either by the Na^+-H^+ exchanger or an H^+-ATPase. This is the active step in the process and results in the accumulation of HCO_3^- in the cytoplasm. This step depends on either the Na^+ gradient established by the Na^+,K^+-ATPase or the pumping of H^+ by an H^+-ATPase. In either case, the cell is alkalinized, allowing more CO_2 to diffuse in. The HCO_3^- moves across the apical membrane in exchange for Cl^-. When H^+ reaches the plasma it combines with HCO_3^- to produce additional CO_2. The rate of HCO_3^- secretion depends on the availability of luminal Cl^-, which is dependent on the

FIGURE 9-1 ■ Model for the secretion of HCO_3^- by the pancreatic duct cell.

opening of the Cl⁻ channel in the apical membrane. This channel is activated by cyclic adenosine monophosphate (cAMP) in response to stimulation by secretin and is present in duct cells but not acinar cells. Na^+ moves down the established electrochemical gradient from the plasma to the lumen of the gland. Water passively moves from the plasma across the cells into the lumen, down the osmotic gradient created by the secretion of Na^+ and HCO_3^-. This secretion is similar to that occurring in the parietal cells of the stomach, except that the H^+ and HCO_3^- are transported in opposite directions. Thus the venous blood from an actively secreting pancreas has a lower pH than that from an inactive gland.

There is new evidence being debated that the bulk of the HCO_3^- entering the cell from the blood may do so via a Na^+-HCO_3^- cotransporter instead of as CO_2.

There is also evidence suggesting that HCO_3 may enter the lumen through a channel, rather than being exchanged for Cl⁻, for it appears that the electrochemical gradient of HCO_3^- established between the lumen and the inside of the ductule cell is sufficient to drive secretion of the ion. This channel may turn out to be the Cl⁻ channel shown in Figure 9-1, which is the CFTR (cystic fibrosis transmembrane conductance regulator) Cl⁻ channel, or a separate anion conductance. This information should be resolved in the near future and, it is hoped, lead to a final revision of the information in Figure 9-1.

As in gastric juice, the ionic concentrations in pancreatic juice vary with the rates of secretion (Figure 9-2). The concentrations of anions (Cl⁻ and HCO_3^-) in pancreatic juice are related inversely to each other, as are the concentrations of cations (Na^+ and H^+) in

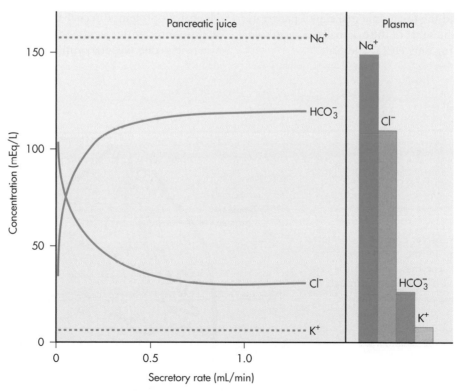

FIGURE 9-2 ■ Relationship between the rate of secretion of pancreatic juice and the concentrations of its major ions. mL/min, milliliters/minute.

gastric juice. Because these relationships are analogous it might be surmised that analogous theories have been proposed to explain them:

- The two-component hypothesis assumes that one cell type, the acinar cell, secretes a small amount of fluid whose major ions are Na^+ and Cl^-. The duct cells secrete large volumes of juice rich in Na^+ and HCO_3^- in response to stimulation. At low rates of secretion, the Cl^- concentration of the juice is therefore relatively high. As the secretory rate increases, the fixed amount of Cl^- being secreted is diluted by the much larger volume of HCO_3^--containing juice, and the final concentrations of the two anions approach those in the pure HCO_3^- secretion.

- Another theory proposes that the cells primarily secrete HCO_3^- and that, as it moves down the ducts, it is exchanged for Cl^-. At low rates of secretion there is sufficient time for the exchange to be nearly complete, and the concentration of each anion is equal to its concentration in plasma. As the rate of secretion increases, less time is available for exchange, and the final ionic makeup of pancreatic juice approaches that of the originally secreted solution containing only HCO_3^- and Na^+.

Both processes probably are involved in determining the final makeup of the secreted juice.

MECHANISMS OF ENZYME SECRETION

The pancreatic acinar cells synthesize and secrete major enzymes for the digestion of all three primary foodstuffs. Like pepsin, the pancreatic proteases are secreted as inactive enzyme precursors and converted to active forms in the lumen. Pancreatic amylase and lipase are secreted in active forms. The activation and specific actions of the pancreatic enzymes are covered in detail in Chapter 11.

Although a certain amount of controversy exists concerning the mechanisms involved in the synthesis and secretion of enzymes by the acinar cells, the process outlined in Figure 9-3 is accepted by most authorities. The secretory process begins with the synthesis of exportable proteins in association with polysomes attached to the cisternae of the rough endoplasmic reticulum (RER) (step 1). As it is being synthesized, the elongating protein, directed by a leader sequence of hydrophobic amino acids, enters the cisternal cavity, where it is collected after synthesis is complete (step 2).

FIGURE 9-3 ■ Pancreatic acinar cell. Note the major steps in the cellular synthesis and secretion of enzymes, and see the text for an explanation of steps 1 through 6. RER, rough endoplasmic reticulum.

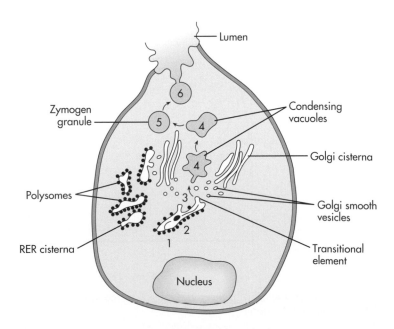

Once within the cisternal space, enzymes remain membrane-bound until they are secreted from the cell. The enzymes next move through the cisternae of the RER to transitional elements, which are associated with smooth vesicles at the Golgi periphery. Possibly as a result of pinching off the transitional elements containing them, the enzymes become associated with the Golgi vesicles (step 3), which transport them to condensing vacuoles (step 4). Energy is required for transport through the endoplasmic reticulum and Golgi vesicles to the condensing vacuoles. Within the condensing vacuoles the enzymes are concentrated to form zymogen granules (step 5). They are then stored in the zymogen granules that collect at the apex of the cell. After a secretory stimulus the membrane of the zymogen granule fuses with the cell membrane, ultimately rupturing and expelling the enzymes into the lumen (step 6). This is the only step in the process that requires a secretory stimulus.

Pancreatic enzymes can also be secreted in the absence of zymogen granules. Enzyme secretion can be maintained at high rates from glands made void of granules by constant stimulation. The mechanism involved in this process, and the interactions between it and the zymogen granule pathway, are not understood.

REGULATION OF SECRETION

As might be expected from its function to neutralize the duodenum, the secretion of fluid and HCO_3^- (the aqueous component) is largely determined by the amount of acid entering the duodenum. The secretion of pancreatic enzymes is similarly determined primarily by the amount of fat and protein entering the duodenum. Control of pancreatic secretion is regulated primarily by secretin, cholecystokinin (CCK), and vagovagal reflexes. Intestinal stimuli account for most pancreatic secretion, but secretion is also stimulated during the cephalic and gastric phases.

Basal pancreatic secretion in humans is low and difficult to measure. The basal secretion of bicarbonate is 2% to 3% of maximal, and basal enzyme secretion is 10% to 15% of maximal. The stimuli for basal secretion are unknown. Because the isolated perfused pancreas secretes basally, this secretion may be an intrinsic property of the gland.

Cephalic Phase

Truncal vagotomy reduces the pancreatic secretory response to a meal by approximately 60%. Most of this decrease is caused by the interruption of vagovagal reflexes and the removal of the potentiating and sensitizing effects of acetylcholine (ACh), which increase the response to secretin. There is, however, a direct vagal component of stimulation that is initiated during the cephalic phase. Sham feeding produces a pancreatic secretory response, which, of course, is blocked totally by vagotomy. In dogs the cephalic phase accounts for approximately 20% of the response to a meal. The stimuli for the cephalic phase of pancreatic secretion are the conditioned reflexes, smell, taste, chewing, and swallowing. Afferent impulses travel to the vagal nucleus. Vagal efferents to the pancreas stimulate both the ductule and the acinar cells to secrete. Stimulation is mediated by ACh and has a greater effect on the enzymatic component than it does on the aqueous component. In dogs a portion of the cephalic phase is mediated by gastrin released by the vagus. Gastrin has about half the potency of CCK for activating the acinar cells. Gastrin plays only a minor role, if any, in the regulation of human pancreatic secretion. These mechanisms are illustrated in Figure 9-4.

Gastric Phase

The stimulation of pancreatic secretion originating from food in the stomach is mediated by the same mechanisms that are involved in the cephalic phase. Distention of the wall of the stomach initiates vagovagal reflexes to the pancreas. Gastrin is released by protein digestion products and distention (see Chapter 8), but again it plays little or no role in the stimulation of the human pancreas.

Intestinal Phase

The presence of digestion products and H^+ in the human small intestine accounts for 70% to 80% of the stimulation of pancreatic secretion. Secretin and CCK account for almost all the hormonal stimulation of pancreatic secretion. The stimulus for the alkaline component (water and bicarbonate) is secretin released from the S cells by gastric acid and high concentrations of long-chain fatty acids. Secretion of the enzymatic component from the acinar cells is

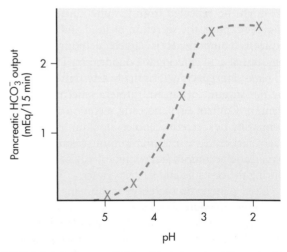

FIGURE 9-4 ■ Mechanisms involved in the stimulation of pancreatic secretion during the cephalic phase. *Dashed lines* represent minor effects. ACh, acetylcholine.

stimulated by CCK released from the I cells by fat and protein digestion products. Current evidence indicates that human acinar cells lack CCK and gastrin receptors. Because vagotomy blocks the secretory response to infusions of physiologic doses of CCK, in humans CCK acts by stimulating vagal afferent receptors and initiating vagovagal reflexes. This stimulation is dependent on cholinergic signaling, for atropine blocks pancreatic secretion in response to CCK. In rodents, acinar cells express CCK receptors and are activated directly by the hormone.

The only potent releaser of secretin is H^+. The duodenal pH threshold for secretin release is 4.5. Secretin release rises almost linearly as the pH is lowered to 3 (Figure 9-5). Lowering the pH below 3 does not lead to greater release of secretin, provided the amount of titratable acid entering the duodenum is held constant. Below pH 3, secretin release and pancreatic

FIGURE 9-5 ■ Pancreatic bicarbonate output in response to various duodenal pH values. The output of bicarbonate is used as an index of secretin release.

bicarbonate secretion are related only to the amount of titratable acid entering the duodenum per unit of time. As more acid enters the gut, more secretin-containing cells are stimulated to release hormone. Thus at a constant pH the amount of secretin released is a function of the length of gut acidified. Secretin can be released from the entire duodenum and jejunum, and the amount of hormone available for release appears to be constant per centimeter (cm) of proximal small intestine.

During the response to a normal meal, however, only the duodenal bulb and proximal duodenum are acidified sufficiently to release secretin. The pH of the proximal duodenum rarely drops below 4 to 3.5. This raises doubts concerning whether sufficient secretin is released by a meal to account for the high rates of pancreatic bicarbonate and water secretion normally seen. If the pH of the gastric contents entering the duodenum is kept at 5 or higher by automatic titration, the pancreatic response is typical of CCK and ACh acting alone (a small volume of enzyme-rich juice). Dropping the pH even slightly below the threshold for secretin release leads to large increases in volume and bicarbonate secretion. The conclusion therefore is that the effects of a small amount of secretin are potentiated by CCK and ACh. In humans, this potentiation is due to ACh alone.

This is an important physiologic interaction of two gastrointestinal (GI) hormones and cholinergic reflexes and is demonstrated directly by the experiment outlined in Figure 9-6. Phenylalanine, a potent releaser of CCK and initiator of vagovagal reflexes, produces a small increase in volume when given alone. If, however, the same dose is infused into the gut while a low dose of secretin is given intravenously, the output of the pancreatic alkaline component increases to levels seen during a meal. Vagotomy greatly decreases the potentiated response. Physiologically, then, in humans, the volume and bicarbonate response to a meal results from small amounts of secretin released by duodenal acidification, being potentiated by ACh from vagovagal reflexes activated by CCK.

Secretin has been referred to as "nature's antacid" because most of its physiologic and pharmacologic actions decrease the amount of acid in the duodenum. For example, it stimulates secretion of HCO_3^- from the pancreas and liver and inhibits gastric secretion and emptying, as well as gastrin release.

FIGURE 9-6 ■ Pancreatic bicarbonate output in response to continual perfusion of the duodenum with phenylalanine, to continuous intravenous infusion of secretin, and to the combination of the two stimuli. Note that the response to secretin is greatly potentiated by endogenous phenylalanine. kg/hr, kilograms/hour.

CCK is the principal humoral regulator of enzyme secretion from the pancreatic acinar cells. It is released in response to amino acids and fatty acids in the small intestine. Only L-isomers of amino acids are effective. In dogs, phenylalanine and tryptophan are potent releasers. Alanine, leucine, and valine are less effective. Phenylalanine, methionine, and valine appear to be potent releasers in humans. CCK is distributed evenly over the first 90 cm of intestine, and infusion of L-phenylalanine below the ligament of Treitz produces pancreatic enzyme responses equal to those seen after infusion near the pylorus. Thus the amount of CCK released depends on the load and length of bowel exposed, as well as on the concentration of amino acids present.

There is strong evidence that some peptides, as well as single amino acids, also release CCK. Three dipeptides, all of which contain glycine (*glycylphenylalanine*, *glycyltryptophan*, and *phenylalanylglycine*), are effective. Dipeptides or tripeptides of glycine, or glycine itself, are ineffective. There is evidence that some peptides containing at least four amino acids are also effective. Undigested protein does not release CCK. After a protein meal, therefore, a wide variety of specific protein products evoke CCK release and pancreatic enzyme secretion.

In addition to protein products, fatty acids longer than eight carbon atoms release CCK and initiate vago-vagal reflexes. *Lauric, palmitic, stearic,* and *oleic acids* are equal and strong releasers of CCK. Fat must be in an absorbable form before release of the hormone occurs. The interactions between luminal nutrients and the receptors triggering the release of CCK, and of GI hormones in general, are poorly understood. As a result, most of the intracellular mechanisms resulting in hormone release are unknown. Part of the reason for this paucity of information has been the inability to isolate large numbers of hormone-containing cells from the mucosa of the GI tract.

Active trypsin in the intestinal lumen inhibits CCK release, and the ingestion of trypsin inhibitors strongly stimulates the release of the hormone. Diversion of pancreatic secretion from the gut lumen also increases plasma CCK. These data suggest the existence of a feedback mechanism controlling the release of CCK. Additional studies indicate that dietary protein products bind or inhibit trypsin, which would otherwise inactivate a CCK-releasing peptide. Several of these peptides have been identified, but their physiologic significance remains to be elucidated.

The mechanisms resulting in the stimulation of pancreatic secretion during the intestinal phase are illustrated in Figure 9-7.

CELLULAR BASIS FOR POTENTIATION

The concept of **potentiation** requires that the potentiating stimuli act on different membrane receptors and trigger different cellular mechanisms for the stimulation

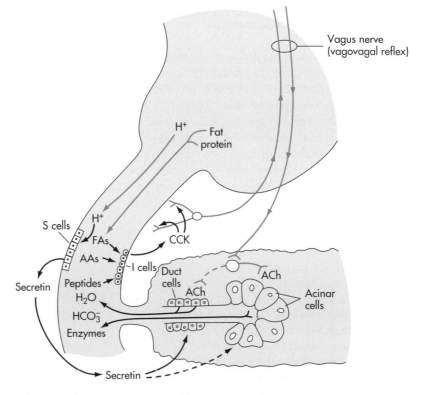

FIGURE 9-7 ■ Mechanisms involved in the stimulation of pancreatic secretion during the intestinal phase in the human. *Dashed lines* indicate potentiative interactions. AAs, amino acids; ACh, acetylcholine; CCK, cholecystokinin; FAs, fatty acids.

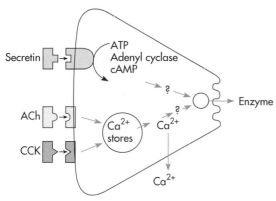

FIGURE 9-8 ■ Receptors on the rodent pancreatic acinar cell. Different second messengers for the stimulants indicate different cellular mechanisms for stimulation and provide the basis for potentiation. ACh, acetylcholine; ATP, adenosine triphosphate; cAMP, cyclic adenosine monophosphate; CCK, cholecystokinin.

of secretion. Some of the steps in these mechanisms have been elucidated for the rodent pancreatic acinar cell; these are illustrated in Figure 9-8.

Secretin binding to its receptor triggers an increase in adenylyl cyclase activity, resulting in the synthesis of cAMP. ACh and CCK bind to separate receptors, but both increase intracellular Ca^{2+}. The Ca^{2+} is mobilized primarily from the plasma membranes and rough endoplasmic reticulum of the acinar cells. Both CCK and ACh also increase diacylglycerol and inositol triphosphate (IP_3) production from phosphatidylinositol. It is likely that one of these breakdown products is the intracellular messenger for Ca^{2+} release. Interactions between secretin and ACh or secretin and CCK result in potentiation. However, the effects of combining CCK and ACh, which trigger identical mechanisms, are only additive. Glucagon and vasoactive intestinal peptide (VIP) also increase cAMP, and gastrin, gastrin-releasing peptide, and substance P increase Ca^{2+} in acinar cells. However, there is no strong evidence that these substances play an important role in the physiologic regulation of pancreatic secretion.

The final steps in the process leading to enzyme secretion have not been elucidated, but they involve the phosphorylation of structural and regulatory proteins. Potentiation occurs because Ca^{2+} and cAMP lead to the activation of different kinases and the phosphorylation of different proteins. The foregoing

interactions have been worked out with guinea pig isolated pancreatic acini. Secretin does not potentiate the effects of CCK and ACh in dogs or humans. A system similar to this, however, is a likely explanation of the potentiation in all species in which it occurs. Thus similar events may be predicted for the human ductule cell, in which secretin (cAMP) is potentiated by ACh (Ca^{2+}).

RESPONSE TO A MEAL

As digestion and mixing of food proceed in the stomach, buffers present in proteins and peptides become saturated with H^+, and the pH drops to about 2. The maximum load of titratable acid (free H^+ plus bound H^+) delivered to the duodenum is 20 to 30 mEq/hour. This is approximately equal to the maximal capacity of the stomach to secrete acid, which, in turn, equals the ability of the pancreas to secrete HCO_3^- when it is maximally stimulated. To raise the pH of the duodenum, the undissociated H^+, as well as the free H^+, must be neutralized. This is accomplished rapidly in the first part of the duodenum, and the pH of the chyme is raised quickly from 2 at the pylorus to above 4 beyond the duodenal bulb. Some neutralization occurs by absorption of H^+ and secretion of HCO_3^- by the gut wall. An additional amount of H^+ is neutralized by HCO_3^- in the bile. The contributions of the gut mucosa and bile, however, are small, and the greatest proportion of acid by far is neutralized by the large volume of pancreatic juice secreted into the lumen.

Within a few minutes after chyme enters the duodenum there is a sharp rise in the secretion of pancreatic enzymes. Within 30 minutes, enzyme secretion peaks at levels about 70% to 80% of those attainable with maximal stimulation by CCK and cholinergic reflexes. Enzyme secretion continues at this rate until the stomach is empty. The enzyme response to a meal may be kept below maximum by the presence of humoral inhibitors of pancreatic secretion. This is the proposed function of pancreatic polypeptide.

Pancreatic enzyme secretion is able to adapt to the diet. In other words, ingestion of a high-protein, low-carbohydrate diet over several days increases the proportion of proteases and decreases the proportion of amylase in pancreatic juice. This type of response is now known to be hormonally regulated at the level of gene expression. CCK increases the expression of the genes for proteases and decreases the expression for amylase. Secretin and gastric inhibitory peptide (GIP) increase the expression of the gene for lipase. The mechanism to increase amylase gene expression under normal conditions is not known, although insulin regulates amylase levels in diabetics.

Insulin potentiates the secretory responses to CCK and secretin, a finding that probably accounts for the reduced pancreatic enzyme secretion in human diabetics who have no obvious pancreatic disease. Insulin also is necessary to maintain normal rates of pancreatic protein synthesis and stores of digestive enzymes.

CLINICAL APPLICATIONS

Abnormal pancreatic secretion occurs with diseases such as chronic and acute pancreatitis, cystic fibrosis, and kwashiorkor, and with tumors that involve the gland itself. Changes in secretion during the course of one of these diseases depend upon the stage of development of the disease. Most patients with **chronic pancreatitis** have decreased volume and bicarbonate output, whereas those with acute pancreatitis often have normal secretion. Both volume and enzyme content of pancreatic juice are decreased by cystic fibrosis. **Tumors of the pancreas** frequently decrease the volume of secretion. With **kwashiorkor,** the alkaline and enzymatic components are depressed, but amylase secretion continues after trypsin, chymotrypsin, and lipase activities are no longer found.

Cystic fibrosis is characterized by decreased Cl^- secretion of many epithelial tissues and the inability of cAMP to regulate Cl^- conductance. As mentioned earlier, there is good evidence that the ion channel for Cl^- in the apical membrane of the duct cell is the cystic fibrosis transmembrane conductance regulator that is regulated by cAMP. Failure to synthesize this protein in its normal state results in cystic fibrosis and a severe decrease of ductal secretion. As a result, proteinaceous acinar secretions become concentrated and precipitate within the duct lumen, blocking small ducts and eventually destroying the gland.

Pancreatic enzyme secretion must be reduced by more than 80% to produce **steatorrhea**. If a patient has steatorrhea, it is only necessary to measure the concentration of any pancreatic enzyme in the jejunal content after a meal to determine whether the condition is pancreatic in origin.

Pancreatic exocrine function is assessed by measuring basal secretion and secretion stimulated by secretin and/or CCK. These function tests are performed on a fasting patient. A double-lumen nasogastric tube is used. One tube opens into the stomach to drain gastric contents that would otherwise empty into the duodenum; the other collects duodenal juice that is assumed to be largely pancreatic in origin. Interpretation of the test is impeded by contaminating biliary secretions. Changes in secretion depend on the stage of development of various diseases and may vary from patient to patient. For these reasons, pancreatic function tests are not reliable in the diagnosis of individual diseases but are used to assess overall pancreatic function.

S U M M A R Y

1. Pancreatic secretion consists of an aqueous bicarbonate component from the duct cells and an enzymatic component from the acinar cells.

2. The duct cells actively secrete HCO_3^- into the lumen, and Na^+ and H_2O follow down electrical and osmotic gradients, respectively.

3. The composition of pancreatic juice varies with the rate of secretion. At low rates Na^+ and Cl^- predominate; at high rates Na^+ and HCO_3^- predominate.

4. Pancreatic enzymes are essential for the digestion of all major foodstuffs and are stored in zymogen granules of acinar cells before secretion.

5. The primary stimulant of the aqueous component is secretin, whose effects are potentiated by CCK and ACh.

6. During the cephalic phase of secretion, vagal stimulation results in a low volume of secretion containing a high concentration of enzymes. This secretion is produced by the acinar cells.

7. During the intestinal phase, acid (with pH less than 4.5) releases secretin. Fats and amino acids release CCK, which activates vagal afferents. The resulting vagovagal reflexes mediated by ACh stimulate enzyme secretion from the acinar cells. Stimulants using different second messengers potentiate each other.

KEY WORDS AND CONCEPTS

- Aqueous component
- Enzymatic/protein component
- Acinar cells
- Ductule cells
- Centroacinar cells
- Islets of Langerhans
- Potentiation
- Chronic pancreatitis
- Tumors of the pancreas
- Kwashiorkor
- Cystic fibrosis
- Steatorrhea

REFERENCES

Anagostides A, Chadwick VS, Selden AC, et al: Sham feeding and pancreatic secretion; Evidence for direct vagal stimulation of enzyme output. Gastroenterology 87:109-114, 1984.

Argent BE, Case RM: Pancreatic ducts: Cellular mechanism and control of bicarbonate secretion. In Johnson LR (ed): Physiology of the Gastrointestinal Tract, 3rd ed. New York, Raven Press, 1994.

Gorelick FS, Jamieson JD: The pancreatic acinar cell: Structure-function relationships. In Johnson LR (ed): Physiology of the Gastrointestinal Tract, 3rd ed. New York, Raven Press, 1994.

Jensen RT: Receptors on pancreatic acinar cells. In Johnson LR (ed): Physiology of the Gastrointestinal Tract, 3rd ed. New York, Raven Press, 1994.

Ji B, Bi Y, Simeone D, et al: Human pancreatic acinar cells lack functional responses to cholecystokinin and gastrin. Gastroenterology 121:1380-1390, 2001.

Logsdon CD: Pancreatic enzyme secretion (physiology). In Johnson LR (ed): Encyclopedia of Gastroenterology vol 3. San Diego, Academic Press, 2004, pp 68-75.

Meyer JH, Way LW, Grossman MI: Pancreatic response to acidification of various lengths of proximal intestine in the dog. Am J Physiol 219:971-977, 1970.

Solomon TE: Control of exocrine pancreatic secretion. In Johnson LR (ed): Physiology of the Gastrointestinal Tract, 3rd ed. New York, Raven Press, 1994.

Solomon TE, Grossman MI: Effect of atropine and vagotomy on response of transplanted pancreas. Am J Physiol 236:E186-E190, 1979.

Yule DI, Williams JA: Stimulus-secretion coupling in the pancreatic acinus. In Johnson LR (ed): Physiology of the Gastrointestinal Tract, 3rd ed. New York, Raven Press, 1994.

10

BILE SECRETION AND GALLBLADDER FUNCTION

NORMAN W. WEISBRODT

Secretion of bile is necessary for the proper digestion and absorption of lipids. It also is required for the normal elimination of various endogenous products (e.g., cholesterol, bile pigments), as well as exogenously administered chemicals (e.g., phenothiazines, heavy metals). Bile secretion is discussed here in three parts: (1) the formation and secretion of bile by the hepatocytes and biliary ducts, (2) the storage and concentration of bile in the gallbladder, and (3) the expulsion and transport of bile from the gallbladder to the lumen of the intestine.

BILE FORMATION

Constituents of Bile

Bile is a complex mixture of organic and inorganic components. Taken separately, some of the components are insoluble and would precipitate out of an aqueous medium. Normally, however, bile is a homogeneous and stable solution whose stability depends on the physical behavior and interactions of its various components.

Bile acids are the major organic constituents of bile, accounting for approximately 50% of the solid components. Chemically they are carboxylic acids with a cyclopentanoperhydrophenanthrene nucleus and a branched side chain of three to nine carbon atoms that ends in a carboxyl group (Figure 10-1). They are related structurally to cholesterol, from which they are synthesized by the liver. Indeed, synthesis of bile acid is a major pathway for the elimination of cholesterol from the body. Conversion of cholesterol to bile acids appears to be via two main synthetic pathways.

The major pathway begins with the rate-limiting step of 7α-hydroxylation of cholesterol by the hepatic enzyme 7α-hydroxylase. A secondary pathway begins with the conversion of cholesterol to 27-hydroxycholesterol, a reaction that takes place in many tissues.

Several features are unique to the bile acids and account for their behavior in solution. Three-dimensionally, the hydroxyl and carboxyl groups are located on one side of the molecule. The bulk of the molecule is composed of the nucleus and several methyl groups (see Figure 10-1). This structure renders bile acids amphipathic to the extent that the hydroxyl and dissociated carboxyl groups are hydrophilic and the nucleus and methyl groupings are hydrophobic. In solution the behavior of bile acids depends on their concentration. At low concentrations there is little interaction among bile acid molecules. As the concentration is increased, a point is reached at which aggregation of the molecules takes place. These aggregates are called **micelles**, and the point of formation is called the **critical micellar concentration**. Hydrophobic regions of the micelles interact with one another, and the hydrophilic regions interact with the water molecules (see Figure 11-13).

The most common human bile acids are cholic acid, chenodeoxycholic acid, deoxycholic acid, and lithocholic acid. These differ from one another primarily in the number of hydroxyl groups present. Cholic acid is a trihydroxy acid; deoxycholic acid and chenodeoxycholic acid are dihydroxy acids; lithocholic acid is a monohydroxy acid and is only slightly soluble.

FIGURE 10-1 ■ Structural formulas for some of the components of bile. On the *left* is a conventional representation. On the *right* is a shorthand version of the Stuart-Briegleb representation. **A,** Cholic acid. Note that the polar hydroxyl groups (the *dark circles*) and the carboxyl group are on the same side of the molecule. **B,** Lecithin. Note that the polar phosphatidylcholine group is at one end and the nonpolar fatty acids are at the other. **C,** Cholesterol. Only one hydroxyl group is present; thus, cholesterol is strongly hydrophobic.

Another feature that affects the aqueous solubility of bile acids is the state of the terminal carboxyl group. The pK of unconjugated bile acids is near neutral; thus, at the pH of intestinal contents they are mostly undissociated and relatively insoluble. In vivo, however, most bile acids exist as conjugates of taurine or glycine.

Conjugated bile acids have much lower pK values and exist as the more soluble dissociated salts at pH values that are found in the biliary tract and intestine.

The second most abundant group of organic compounds in bile is the **phospholipids,** the major ones being the lecithins (see Figure 10-1). Phospholipids also are amphipathic, insofar as the phosphatidylcholine grouping is hydrophilic, whereas the fatty acid chains are hydrophobic. Although amphipathic, the phospholipids are not soluble in water but form liquid crystals that swell in solution. In the presence of bile salts, however, the liquid crystals are broken up and solubilized as a component of the micelles. Bile salts possess a large capacity to solubilize phospholipids; 2 moles (mol) of lecithin are solubilized by 1 mol of bile salts. The combination of bile salts and phospholipids also is better able to solubilize other lipids—mainly cholesterol— than is a simple solution of bile salts.

A third organic component, **cholesterol**, is present in small amounts, contributing about 4% to the total solids of bile. Although present in small amounts, bile cholesterol is important because it may be excreted and therefore helps regulate body stores of cholesterol. Cholesterol appears mainly in the nonesterified form and is insoluble in water. In the presence of bile salts and phospholipids, however, it is solubilized as part of the micelle. Because it is a weakly polar substance, cholesterol is found in the interior of the micelle, where the hydrophobic portions of the bile salts and phospholipids interact.

The fourth major group of organic compounds found in bile is the **bile pigments**. These constitute only 2% of the total solids, with bilirubin being the most important. Chemically, bile pigments are tetrapyrroles and are related to the porphyrins, from which they are derived. In their free form, bile pigments are insoluble in water. Normally, however, they are conjugated with glucuronic acid and rendered soluble. Unlike the other organic compounds just mentioned, bile pigments do not take part in micellar formation. As their name implies, they are highly colored substances. Other than being responsible for the normal color of bile and feces, the pigment properties of these compounds are used to assess the level of function of the liver.

In addition to the organic compounds just discussed, many **inorganic ions** are found in bile. The predominant cation is Na^+, accompanied by smaller amounts of K^+ and Ca^{++}. The predominant inorganic anions are Cl^- and HCO_3^-. Normally the total number of inorganic cations will exceed the total number of inorganic anions. There is no anion deficit, however, because the bile acids, which possess a net negative charge at the pH values

found in bile, account for the difference. Bile is isosmotic even though there is a larger than expected number of cations present. Because they are highly charged molecules, the bile acids attract a layer of cations that serve as counterions. These counterions are tightly associated with the micelles and thus exert little osmotic activity. Therefore, bile is isosmotic even though the number of cations present is larger than expected.

BILE SECRETION

The secretion of bile depends heavily on the secretion of bile acids by the liver. Once secreted, bile acids undergo an interesting journey (Figure 10-2). First, they may be stored in the **gallbladder**. Then they are propelled into and through the small intestine, where they take part in the digestion and absorption of lipids. Most of the bile acids themselves are absorbed from the intestine and travel via the portal blood to the liver, where they are taken up by the hepatocytes and resecreted. This process is termed **enterohepatic circulation**.

Bile acids are secreted continuously by the **liver**. The rate of secretion, however, varies widely. Early experiments demonstrated that the rate of secretion depended on the amount of bile acids delivered to the liver via the blood; the more acids in the portal blood, the greater the secretion of bile. The amount of bile acids in the portal blood depends on the amount absorbed from the small intestine. The amount of bile acids in the intestine, in turn, depends on the digestive state of the individual. Between meals, most bile secreted by the liver is stored in the gallbladder, with only small amounts being delivered intermittently to the small intestine. During a meal the gallbladder empties its contents into the duodenum in a more continuous pattern. The ejected bile acids are then resorbed from the intestine and resecreted by the liver. It is estimated that the total amount of bile acids in the body is secreted twice during the digestion of each meal.

Although a wide variety of bile acids are found in the bile, only cholic and chenodeoxycholic acids appear to be synthesized from cholesterol in significant amounts by human hepatocytes. For this reason they are called "primary" bile acids. Their synthesis by the liver is a continuous but regulated process. The amount synthesized depends on the amount of bile acids

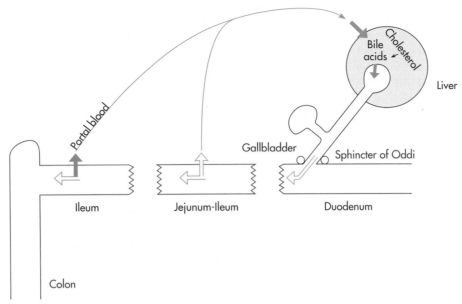

FIGURE 10-2 ■ Enterohepatic circulation of bile acids. Bile acids are actively secreted by the liver. Once in the intestine they participate in the digestion and absorption of lipids. As they are propelled toward the distal small bowel, some of the "primary" acids are altered, becoming "secondary" acids. The more hydrophobic bile acids are absorbed passively throughout the intestine. The more hydrophilic acids are absorbed by a sodium-coupled active transport process that is localized to the ileum. A minor fraction of bile acids is not absorbed but is instead propelled into the colon. The absorbed bile acids are transported via the portal circulation to the liver, where they are extracted actively from the blood (at a rate of almost 100%) and resecreted. Synthesis of new primary acids from cholesterol occurs at a rate to compensate for the acids lost from the bowel. *Solid arrows* denote active absorption, secretion, and synthesis; *open arrows* denote passive absorption and propulsion of contents by contractions of the intestine.

returned to the liver in the enterohepatic circulation. If most of the bile acids secreted by the liver are returned, synthesis is low, but if the secreted acids are lost from the enterohepatic circulation, the rate of synthesis is high. Normally there are 1 to 2 grams (g) of bile salts in the enterohepatic circulation. If the absorptive processes in the intestine and liver are functioning properly, only about 0.5 g is lost daily. Synthesis is regulated to replenish this loss.

Deoxycholic acid, lithocholic acid, and other "secondary" bile acids are produced in the intestine through the action of microorganisms on primary bile acids. These acids then are absorbed along with the primary bile acids, taken up by the **hepatocytes**, conjugated with taurine and glycine, and secreted in the bile. Thus bile contains a mixture of primary and secondary bile acids. Cholic, chenodeoxycholic, and deoxycholic

acids normally appear in a ratio of 4:4:2. Usually only a small amount of lithocholic acid is present.

The enterohepatic circulation of bile acids is characterized by both passive and active transport processes (see Figure 10-2). The more hydrophobic bile acids—those with fewer hydroxyl groups and those that become deconjugated—are absorbed passively throughout the intestine. The more hydrophilic acids are absorbed by an active process that is localized to the ileum. Uptake across the apical membrane of the enterocytes is mediated by a specific sodium-dependent transporter protein. Transport through the cell to the basolateral membrane is mediated by binding proteins. Transport across the basolateral membrane out of the cell is mediated by a sodium-independent anion exchange process that involves a carrier different from the one on the apical membrane. As stated previously, the ileal transport process is highly efficient, delivering greater than 90% of the bile acids to the portal blood. In the liver, a second transport process removes bile acids from the portal blood. In large part, uptake into hepatocytes is mediated by a sodium-dependent transporter protein that shares similarities with, but is distinct from, the ileal transporter. In addition, there are other organic anion-transporting polypeptides that mediate the uptake of not only bile acids but also other large anionic molecules. Transport of bile acids through the hepatocytes to the canalicular membrane is mediated by a number of binding proteins. At the canaliculus, bile acids and other organic anions appear to be secreted by one or more adenosine triphosphate (ATP)-dependent processes. The hepatic transport of bile acids also is highly efficient. Practically all bile acids contained in the portal blood are removed during one passage through the liver. The process does have a transport maximum, but this is seldom reached.

Cholesterol and phospholipids, primarily lecithins, also are secreted by the hepatocytes. The exact mechanisms of secretion are not known, but secretion appears to depend, in part, on the secretion of bile acids. The higher the rate of bile acid secretion, the higher the rate of cholesterol and phospholipid secretion. Once secreted into the intestine along with the other components of bile, cholesterol and lecithin are mixed with

and handled as ingested cholesterol and lecithin (see Chapter 11).

The primary bile pigment in humans, **bilirubin**, is derived largely from the metabolic breakdown of **hemoglobin** (Figure 10-3). Most of the hemoglobin comes from aged red blood cells (RBCs) that are disposed of by cells of the reticuloendothelial (RE) system. In the RE cells, hemoglobin is split into hemin and globin. The hemin ring is opened and oxidized, and the iron is removed to form bilirubin, which is then transported via the blood from the cells of the RE system to the hepatocytes. In transit, bilirubin is tightly bound to plasma albumin; very little is free in the plasma. Hepatocytes possess the ability to extract bilirubin from blood, conjugate it with glucuronic acid, and secrete the conjugated product into the bile. Bilirubin secretion into the bile by the hepatocytes is mediated by an active anion transport system. This system is different from the one for active transport of bile acids, but it is shared by a number of other organic anions (e.g., sulfobromophthalein [Bromsulphalein, or BSP], various radiopaque dyes).

Bilirubin is not absorbed from the intestine in any appreciable amount. Some of the product, however, is altered in the bowel. Bacteria, primarily in the distal small bowel and colon, reduce bilirubin to urobilinogen, which is unconjugated. Some urobilinogen is

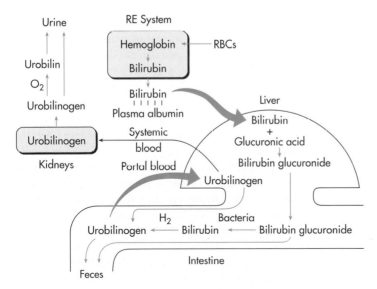

FIGURE 10-3 ■ Excretion of bile pigments. Bilirubin is produced by cells of the reticuloendothelial system from aged red blood cells. The unconjugated pigment is then carried, tightly bound to plasma albumin, to the liver. There it is actively taken up, conjugated with glucuronic acid, and secreted into the bile. The water-soluble conjugates are propelled along the intestine. In the distal small bowel and colon a portion of the conjugated pigment is acted on by bacteria and becomes unconjugated bilirubin and other pigments. Some of these pigments are absorbed passively into the blood and either returned to the liver and resecreted or passed through the liver and excreted by the kidneys. Most, however, pass through the colon and are excreted. **Bold arrows** indicate active absorption. RBCs, red blood cells; RE, reticuloendothelial.

converted to stercobilin and is excreted in the feces. Urobilinogen also is absorbed into the portal blood and returned to the liver. There most is extracted, conjugated, and secreted into the bile; however, some passes into the systemic circulation and is excreted by the kidneys. The urobilinogen is oxidized in the urine to form urobilin. Stercobilin and urobilin are pigments that are in large part responsible for the color of the feces and urine, respectively.

Two components of bile water and electrolyte secretion have been identified. One is called **bile acid–dependent secretion**. Bile acids, regardless of whether they are newly synthesized or extracted from the portal blood, are the major component actively secreted by the hepatocytes. Because they are anions, their secretion is accompanied by the passive movement of cations into the canaliculus which in turn sets up an osmotic gradient down which water moves (Figure 10-4). The second component is called **bile acid–independent secretion**. There is evidence for the active transport of Na^+ by the hepatocytes. Also, as the canalicular bile flows through the bile ductules and ducts on its way to the gallbladder, its composition is altered (see Figure 10-4). Both secretion and absorption take place in the ducts, with secretion normally predominating. Bicarbonate is actively secreted by the epithelial cells that line the ducts. Both secretion and absorption of Na^+, Cl^-, and water also can be demonstrated. The net effect of this secretory and absorptive activity is that the bile becomes more alkaline, and its chloride content decreases. Secretory activity of the epithelial cells of the bile ductules and ducts is under hormonal control. Secretin stimulates production of bile that is relatively low in bile salt and high in HCO_3^- concentration. It does this by increasing the active transport of sodium and bicarbonate from the epithelial cells into the bile.

BILE TRANSPORT TO AND STORAGE IN THE GALLBLADDER

The force responsible for the flow of bile from the canaliculi toward the small intestine is primarily the secretory pressure generated by the hepatocytes and ductule epithelium. The hepatic end of the biliary tract is blind, being formed by the secretory cells of the liver. Thus, as bile is secreted by these cells, pressure in

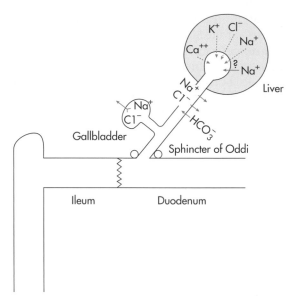

FIGURE 10-4 ■ Secretion and absorption of water and electrolytes. The osmotic gradient created by the active secretion of bile acids, and perhaps Na^+, causes water to move from the hepatocytes into the bile canaliculi. Ions accompany water movement, presumably via the process of bulk flow. Epithelial cells of the bile ducts are capable of actively absorbing Na^+ and Cl^- and of actively secreting Na^+ and HCO_3^-. In the gallbladder, salt absorption is accompanied by the absorption of water, thus concentrating the bile.

the ducts rises. The active secretion of bile acids and electrolytes can make biliary secretory pressures reach a level of 10 to 20 millimeters of mercury (mm Hg).

Whether bile flows into the duodenum or into the gallbladder depends on a balance between resistance to the filling of the gallbladder and resistance to bile flowing through the terminal **bile duct** and **sphincter of Oddi.** The gallbladder is a distensible muscular organ that forms a blind outpouching of the biliary tract. Its inner surface is lined with a thin layer of epithelial cells having high absorptive capacity. The sphincter of Oddi is a thickening of the circular muscle of the bile duct located at the ductal entrance into the duodenum. Although this muscle is embedded in the wall of the duodenum, it appears to be an entity separate from the duodenal musculature. Most of the time during fasting, the gallbladder is readily distensible, and the sphincter of Oddi maintains closure of the terminal bile duct.

Thus, bile secreted by the liver flows into the gallbladder (Figure 10-5A).

The human gallbladder is not a large organ and when full can accommodate only 20 to 50 milliliters (mL) of fluid. During fasting, however, many times that volume of fluid may be secreted by the liver. The discrepancy between the amount of bile secreted by the liver and the amount stored in the gallbladder is accounted for by the gallbladder's ability to concentrate bile. The concentration of bile salts, bile pigments, and other large water-soluble molecules may increase by a factor of 5 to 20 as a result of water and electrolyte absorption.

Absorption of water and electrolytes is partly an active process. Na$^+$ absorption can occur against an electro-chemical gradient, is a saturable process, depends on metabolic activity, and demonstrates other character-istics of an active transport mechanism. Unlike the transport mechanisms for Na$^+$ that exist in other epithelia, however, transport in the gallbladder is not associated with generation of any measurable electrical potential difference. In addition, it is highly dependent on the presence of either Cl$^-$ or HCO$_3^-$. Thus, it appears as if Na$^+$ transport is coupled with the transport of an anion and is electrically neutral.

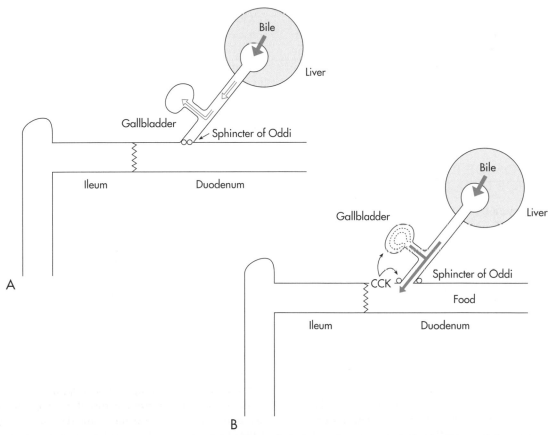

FIGURE 10-5 ■ **A,** Bile flow between periods of digestion. Bile is secreted continuously by the liver and flows toward the duodenum. In the interdigestive period the gallbladder is readily distensible, and the sphincter of Oddi is contracted. Therefore bile flows into the gallbladder rather than the duodenum. **B,** On eating, both hormonal (e.g., cholecystokinin [CCK]) and neural stimuli cause contraction of the gallbladder and relaxation of the sphincter of Oddi. Thus, bile flows into the bowel. Bile secretion from the liver increases as bile acids are returned via the enterohepatic circulation.

As in other epithelial tissue, water movement in the gallbladder is dependent on the active absorption of NaCl and NaHCO$_3$, and thus it is entirely passive. The rows of epithelial cells of the mucosa have large lateral intercellular spaces near the basal membrane and possess tight junctions at cell apices. Solute is transported actively from the cells into the intercellular space at the apical ends. This movement is then followed by the passive diffusion of H$_2$O. The movement of water molecules, however, is such that an osmotic gradient is set up in the intercellular spaces. The solution is hypertonic at the apical end and isotonic at the basal end. In the steady state, this standing osmotic gradient is maintained and accounts for the absorption of a solution with fixed osmolality.

Absorption of Na$^+$, Cl$^-$, HCO$_3^-$, and H$_2$O influences the concentrations of other solutes in the bile. Ions such as K$^+$ and Ca^{++} become more concentrated. The concentration of bile salts also increases during the absorption of water and electrolytes, often to the point of the critical micellar concentration. The presence of micelles, which have minimal osmotic activity, permits the high concentration of electrolytes, bile salts, phospholipids, and cholesterol to be isotonic in gallbladder bile.

EXPULSION OF BILE AND TRANSPORT TO THE INTESTINE

Most bile secretion occurs during the digestion of meals. However, significant amounts are secreted periodically during fasting in synchrony with the migrating motor complex (MMC) (see pp. 36-37, 43). The gallbladder contracts, expelling bile, shortly before and during the period of intense sequential duodenal contractions. Thus bile, along with other secretions, is swept aborally along the bowel by these contractions. The exact stimuli and pathways responsible for coordinating gallbladder contraction with cyclic intestinal motility are not known, but they appear to involve cholinergic nerves.

Shortly after eating, the gallbladder musculature contracts rhythmically and empties gradually (Figure 10-5B). The stimulus for its contraction appears to be primarily hormonal. Products of food digestion, particularly lipids, release **cholecystokinin** (CCK) from the mucosa of the duodenum. This hormone is carried in the blood to the gallbladder, where it stimulates the musculature to contract. CCK is a stimulant of gallbladder muscle and may act in part by binding to receptors located directly on smooth muscle cells. In vivo, however, much of CCK's action appears to be mediated through extrinsic vagal and intrinsic cholinergic nerves. The role of other gastrointestinal (GI) hormones is less clear. Gastrin stimulates gallbladder contraction, but in doses that are well above the physiologic range. Secretin appears to have little direct effect on the gallbladder, although it may antagonize (or prevent) the effects of CCK. Pancreatic polypeptide and somatostatin both have been shown to decrease gallbladder contractility and may affect gallbladder function in certain disease states.

The flow of bile from the gallbladder through the common bile duct and into the duodenum is influenced by muscular activity of the common bile duct, sphincter of Oddi, and duodenum. The bile duct contains smooth muscle cells, and measurements of its contractile activity have been made in certain species. Some investigators maintain that peristaltic contractions of the duct do occur, and that these facilitate movement of bile into the duodenum. The relative importance of this mechanism is not known.

The sphincter of Oddi is a muscular ring surrounding the opening of the bile duct in the wall of the duodenum. Its relative contributions to the regulation of bile flow sometimes are difficult to assess because its own activity is influenced by the musculature of the duodenum. The sphincter can maintain closure of the bile duct independently of activity of the duodenal musculature. When the duodenum is relaxed, pressures of 12 to 30 mm Hg are needed to force fluid through a closed sphincter. However, bile flow through an open sphincter of Oddi is influenced markedly by the contractile activity of the duodenum. Bile enters an actively contracting bowel in spurts during periods of duodenal relaxation and stops during periods of contraction. The sphincter, like the muscle of the gallbladder, is controlled by the hormone CCK. In contrast with its action on the gallbladder, CCK relaxes the sphincter of Oddi and thereby allows bile to enter the duodenum. In a manner similar to its mechanism of action on the gallbladder, CCK appears to influence sphincter of Oddi function by acting on nerves, rather than directly on smooth muscle.

The role of the autonomic nervous system (ANS) in the control of bile flow is not clear. Stimulation of parasympathetic nerves causes an increase in bile flow and contraction of the gallbladder. Stimulation of sympathetic nerves has the opposite effect. Bile flow begins shortly after eating and may be part of the cephalic phase of digestion. The emotional state of the person also has been shown to influence bile flow.

CLINICAL APPLICATIONS

Abnormalities of bile secretion can result from functional changes in the liver, bile ducts, gallbladder, and intestine. Because many of the components of bile are synthesized and/or actively secreted by hepatocytes, metabolic abnormalities of these cells can result in decreased bile production and increased plasma levels of those constituents normally excreted in the bile (e.g., bile acids, bile pigments). Metabolic abnormalities more commonly result from the destruction of hepatocytes by infectious agents (e.g., viral hepatitis) and various toxins. There are, however, several conditions characterized by genetic deficiencies in one or more of the steps of bilirubin secretion. These deficiencies also can result in **jaundice** (a visually detectable buildup of bile pigments in the blood).

Besides the rather striking changes in hepatocyte function seen with hepatocyte destruction and genetic defects, subtle changes also can produce pathologic conditions. In many individuals, the quantity of bile produced by the liver may be normal, but the quality may be abnormal. To be stable, bile must contain certain proportions of bile salts, phospholipids, and cholesterol. If there is a relative excess of cholesterol, it may precipitate to form gallstones.

Abnormalities of the bile ducts and gallbladder usually are secondary to the processes of obstruction (e.g., stones, tumor) and infection. **Obstruction** can result in severe pain and lead to reflux of bile into the liver parenchyma and eventually the systemic circulation. **Bacterial infections,** often occurring secondary to stones, also can initiate and/or perpetuate stone formation. Several strains of bacteria (such as *Escherichia coli*) produce β-glucuronidase, which deconjugates conjugated bile pigments. These unconjugated pigments, which are less soluble, then precipitate to form pigment stones or a nidus for precipitation of cholesterol.

Abnormalities of intestinal function can alter the secretion of products that undergo enterohepatic circulation. For example, if the terminal ileum is diseased or removed, bile salt absorption is reduced. This decreases the bile salt pool (and hence bile salt secretion) and increases synthesis of bile acids by the liver. In addition, bile acids that enter the colon induce water secretion by the colonic mucosa, causing diarrhea.

CLINICAL TESTS

The major tests of bile secretion revolve around measurement of serum levels of endogenous substances normally secreted in the bile, measurement of secretion of exogenous substances injected into the blood, and x-ray, scintigraphic, and ultrasonographic visualizations of the biliary tract.

Plasma levels of both bile salts and bile pigments are elevated in many types of hepatobiliary disease. Of these substances, bilirubin is the most commonly measured entity. Abnormalities in hepatic function often can be detected before the elevation of serum bilirubin and the development of jaundice. This is done by intravenously injecting chemicals such as sulfobromophthalein and indocyanine green. These substances normally are taken up and secreted by the same anionic transport system used for the hepatic secretion of bile pigments. Impairment of hepatocyte function is characterized by a slower than normal disappearance of these injected substances from the blood.

Many **gallstones** are radiopaque and can be visualized on a plain abdominal x-ray film. Others, however, are radiolucent and thus not obvious; a radiopaque dye is required to facilitate visualization of these stones. The dye usually consists of iodinated anions that are taken up and secreted by the anionic transport system of the hepatocytes. The stones are then surrounded by the dye and appear as holes in the contrast medium. Radiopaque dyes are effective only if the anionic transport system of the hepatocytes is functional; therefore, the tests do not work in the presence of jaundice. Scintigraphy and especially ultrasound examination are becoming routine for the confirmation or exclusion of gallstone disease. Ultrasonography can provide information about the thickness of the gallbladder wall, the presence of intramural gas, and even the diameter of intrahepatic and extrahepatic bile ducts.

SUMMARY

1. Bile is secreted by the liver as a complex mixture of bile acids, phospholipids, cholesterol, bile pigments, electrolytes, and water.

2. Primary bile acids are synthesized from cholesterol by the hepatocytes and conjugated to taurine and glycine. Conjugated bile acids are amphipathic and, along with phospholipids and cholesterol, form mixed micelles in aqueous solution at pH values found in the intestine. Micelles take part in the digestion and absorption of dietary lipids and lipid-soluble substances.

3. Hepatic bile secretion depends primarily on the secretion of bile acids. Bile acid secretion in turn depends on hepatocyte uptake of bile acids from the portal blood and on bile acid synthesis. Bile secretion depends to a lesser degree on electrolyte secretion by hepatocytes and ductule cells.

4. During the fasting state, most secreted bile is stored in the gallbladder, where electrolytes and water are absorbed, thus concentrating the bile acids as an isosmotic micellar solution. Small amounts of bile empty into the duodenum during the MMC.

5. During the fed state, the gallbladder contracts, thereby expelling larger quantities of bile into the duodenum. Gallbladder contraction is due mostly to the action of CCK released from the upper intestine in response to food products.

6. In the intestine some bile acids are deconjugated, and some primary bile acids are dehydroxylated to form secondary bile acids. These, along with the still-conjugated primary bile acids, are absorbed from the intestine either passively along the length of intestine or actively through a sodium-coupled transport process in the ileum. Once absorbed into the portal circulation, bile acids are returned to the liver, where they are actively absorbed by a sodium-coupled transport process, conjugated (if need be), and resecreted. This pattern of bile acid secretion, absorption, and resecretion is termed the enterohepatic circulation.

KEY WORDS AND CONCEPTS

- Bile
- Bile acids
- Micelles
- Critical micellar concentration
- Phospholipids
- Cholesterol
- Bile pigments
- Inorganic ions
- Gallbladder
- Enterohepatic circulation
- Liver
- Hepatocytes
- Bilirubin
- Hemoglobin
- Bile acid–dependent secretion
- Bile acid–independent secretion
- Bile duct
- Sphincter of Oddi
- Cholecystokinin
- Jaundice
- Obstruction
- Bacterial infections
- Gallstones

REFERENCES

Dawson P, Shneider B, Hofmann A: Bile formation and the enterohepatic circulation. In Johnson LR (ed): Physiology of the Gastrointestinal Tract, 4th ed. San Diego, Elsevier, 2006.

Mawe GM, Saccone TP, Pozo MJ: Neural control of the gallbladder and sphincter of Oddi. In Johnson LR (ed): Physiology of the Gastrointestinal Tract, 4th ed. San Diego, Elsevier, 2006.

Moseley RH: Bile secretion. In Yamada T, Alpers DH, Laine L, et al (eds): Textbook of Gastroenterology, vol 1, 3rd ed. Philadelphia, Lippincott Williams & Wilkins, 1999.

Scharschmidt BF: Bilirubin metabolism, bile formation, and gallbladder and bile duct function. In Sleisenger MH, Fordtran JS (eds): Gastrointestinal Disease, vol 2, 5th ed. Philadelphia, WB Saunders, 1993.

11

DIGESTION AND ABSORPTION

LEONARD R. JOHNSON

M otility and secretion are regulated to ensure the efficient digestion of food and absorption of nutrients across the mucosa of the gastrointestinal (GI) tract. This chapter explains how food is broken down into small absorbable molecules and how these products are transported into the blood.

STRUCTURAL-FUNCTIONAL ASSOCIATIONS

Food assimilation takes place primarily in the small intestine and is aided by anatomic modifications that increase the luminal surface area—Kerckring's folds, villi, and microvilli. The microvilli are prominent on the apical surface of columnar epithelial cells or enterocytes and occur to a lesser extent on goblet cells. Collectively the microvillous regions constitute the **brush border.**

Several cell types make up the intestinal epithelium. Students of digestive and absorptive physiology are most familiar with **enterocytes** and **goblet cells.** Enterocytes function in digestion, absorption, and secretion. Goblet cells secrete mucus. The function of mucus is not clear but may be related to physical, chemical, and immunologic protection. Both enterocytes and goblet cells are derived from a common stem cell within the intestinal crypts. Enterocytes and goblet cells become differentiated as they move upward from the base of the crypt, and their characteristics are expressed more strongly as they migrate farther up the villus. As they reach the tip of the villus the cells are extruded and become

a component of the succus entericus. In humans the time needed to replace the entire population of epithelial cells (the cell turnover time) is 3 to 6 days. Cell proliferation, differentiation, and maturation are influenced by GI hormones, growth factors, other endocrine substances, and the nature of the material in the lumen. These processes are also altered by starvation, irradiation, and the loss of a portion of the bowel. The rapid proliferative rate of the intestinal mucosa makes it vulnerable to radiation and chemotherapy, procedures used to treat cancer. Despite the interplay between a basic dynamic process and the extrinsic factors that affect epithelial development, under normal conditions the mucosal appearance remains relatively constant.

DIGESTION

Digestion is the chemical breakdown of food by enzymes secreted by glandular cells in the mouth, chief cells in the stomach, and the exocrine cells of the pancreas, or enzymes bound to the apical membranes of enterocytes. Although some digestion of carbohydrates, proteins, and fats takes place in the stomach, the final breakdown of these substances occurs in the small intestine.

The enzymes important in digestion are summarized in Figure 11-1. **Luminal** or **cavital digestion** is due to enzymes secreted by the salivary glands, stomach, and pancreas. Significant chemical degradation of food is also carried out by hydrolytic enzymes associated with the small intestinal brush border. Hydrolysis by these

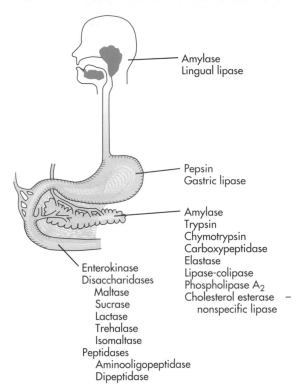

Amylase
Lingual lipase

Pepsin
Gastric lipase

Amylase
Trypsin
Chymotrypsin
Carboxypeptidase
Elastase
Lipase-colipase
Phospholipase A$_2$
Cholesterol esterase —
   nonspecific lipase

Enterokinase
Disaccharidases
  Maltase
  Sucrase
  Lactase
  Trehalase
  Isomaltase
Peptidases
  Aminooligopeptidase
  Dipeptidase

FIGURE 11-1 ■ Source of the principal luminal and membrane-bound digestive enzymes.

enzymes is termed **contact** or **membrane digestion.** *Membrane digestion* is a more acceptable term, because *contact digestion* connotes activity by exogenous enzymes that become adsorbed on the epithelial surface. Membrane digestion refers to hydrolysis by enzymes synthesized by epithelial cells and inserted into the apical membrane as integral components. The half-life of membrane-bound enzymes (such as oligosaccharidases) is shorter than that of the epithelial cells. Thus, breakdown and resynthesis occur several times during the life of a single cell.

Digestion and absorption of essentially all major dietary products take place in the small intestine. Despite the degradation of colonic contents by bacteria, physiologically important digestion does not occur in the colon. Nonetheless, absorption in this organ is impressive. A practical illustration is that some medications administered as rectal suppositories are systemically

functional. During periods of health the principal substances absorbed from the colon are water and electrolytes. However, life is possible without this organ, as evidenced by patients who thrive after colectomy.

ABSORPTION

Although the brush border is the site of activity for a number of digestive enzymes, it is also the barrier that must be traversed by nutrients, water, and electrolytes on the way to the blood or lymph. The terms *transport* and *absorption* often are used interchangeably to mean the movement of materials from the intestinal lumen into the blood. *Secretion* implies movement in the opposite direction.

Mucosal Membrane

Conceptually the plasma membrane of the enterocyte is often considered the only factor restricting the free movement of substances from the gut lumen into the blood or lymph. However, transmural movement actually takes place over a complex pathway. This is conveyed schematically in Figure 11-2 and includes (1) an **unstirred layer of fluid,** (2) the **glycocalyx** ("fuzzy coat") covering the microvilli, (3) the cell membrane, (4) the cytoplasm of the enterocyte, (5) the basal or lateral cell membrane, (6) the intercellular space, (7) the basement membrane, and (8) the membrane of the capillary or lymph vessel.

Transport Processes

An outstanding property of the enterocyte membrane is its capacity to control the flux of solutes and fluid between the lumen and blood. This involves several mechanisms. Pinocytosis occurs at the base of microvilli and may be a major mechanism in the uptake of protein. Other uptake processes include **passive diffusion, facilitated diffusion,** and **active transport.** In the case of passive diffusion, the epithelium behaves like an inert barrier, and the particles traverse this cell layer through pores in the cell membrane or through intercellular spaces. Lipid-soluble substances can diffuse through lipid portions of the membrane. The tight junction between apposing enterocytes (see Figure 11-2) forms a mechanical seal that prevents mixing of interstitial fluid with luminal contents. This seal, however,

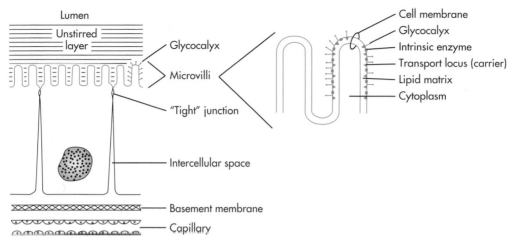

FIGURE 11-2 ■ Mucosal barrier. Solutes moving across the enterocyte from the intestinal lumen to the blood must traverse an unstirred layer of fluid, a glycocalyx, the apical membrane, the cytoplasm of the cell, the basolateral cell membrane, the basement membrane, and finally the wall of the capillary of the lymphatic vessel. Microvilli are morphologic modifications of the cell membrane that comprise the brush border. The importance of this region in the digestion and absorption of nutrients is depicted by the enlarged microvillus, which illustrates the spatial arrangement of enzymes and carrier molecules.

is relatively leaky to ions and water in certain regions of the intestine, allowing some exchange between the lumen and intercellular spaces.

ADAPTATION OF DIGESTIVE AND ABSORPTIVE PROCESSES

Alterations in intestinal functions in response to a variety of factors are well documented. Functional adjustments that maintain homeostasis or allow an animal to cope better with its environment are termed *adaptations*. The quality and degree of adjustment are dependent upon the type of environmental stimulus encountered. Clinical situations in which the capacity to adapt is magnified are small-bowel resection and bypass. Until recently physicians knew only that a patient subjected to one of these operations underwent an initial phase of undernutrition, steatorrhea, and acidic diarrhea, and that these symptoms tended to be alleviated with time. Relief from the symptoms is believed to be attributable to adaptations. For example, after proximal bowel resection or bypass, the remaining segment undergoes hyperplastic changes accompanied by enhancement of particular absorptive and digestive functions. Adaptation is limited in

some circumstances. This point is illustrated by the fact that the carrier-mediated absorption of vitamin B_{12} and bile salts is confined strictly to the terminal ileum. Other regions of the GI tract cannot compensate if the absorptive capacity for these compounds in the ileum is lost.

With certain genetic abnormalities, such as lactase deficiency, the capacity to adapt is lost. Lactase deficiency and also pancreatic and intestinal diseases of varied etiology contribute to maldigestion and malabsorption.

CARBOHYDRATE ASSIMILATION

Principal Dietary Forms

The average daily intake of carbohydrates, which account for approximately 50% of the calories ingested, is about 300 grams (g) in the United States. **Starch** comprises about 50% of the total, **sucrose** about 30%, **lactose** 6%, and **maltose** 1% to 2%. Trehalose, glucose, fructose, sorbitol, cellulose, hemicellulose, and pectins make up most of the remainder. Starch is a high-molecular-weight compound consisting of two polysaccharides, amylose and amylopectin. Amylose is a straight-chain polymer of glucose linked by α-1,4- glycosidic bonds. The repeating disaccharide unit is maltose. **Amylopectin,** a plant starch, is the major form of carbohydrate in the diet and is similar to amylose; however, in addition to 1,4- linkages there is a 1,6- linkage for every 20 to 30 glucose units. Glycogen is a high-molecular-weight polysaccharide similar to amylopectin in molecular structure but having considerably more 1,6- linkages. Maltose and trehalose are dimers of glucose in 1,4- and 1,1- linkages, respectively. Sucrose is a disaccharide consisting of 1 mole (mol) of glucose bound at the number 1 carbon to the number 2 carbon of fructose. Lactose is 1 mol of galactose bound at the number 1 carbon to the number 4 carbon of glucose in a β-linkage.

Digestion

Luminal digestion of starch begins in the mouth with the action of salivary α-amylase and ends in the small intestine through the action of pancreatic α-amylase, which is 94% homologous to salivary amylase. Human salivary and pancreatic amylases have optimum activities near neutral pH and are activated by Cl⁻. Although salivary amylase is destroyed by acid in the stomach, some enzymatic activity occurs within the bolus of food. Most starch digestion, however, occurs in the small intestine. Hydrolysis occurs not only in the lumen but also at the surface of epithelial cells because some amylase is adsorbed to the brush border.

Amylase attacks only the interior α-1,4- bonds of amylose, yielding maltose and the trisaccharide maltotriose. Hydrolysis of amylopectin and glycogen yields similar products plus α-limit dextrins (Figure 11-3). The latter are oligosaccharides of glucose, formed because the α-1,6- linkages and the α-1,4- bonds near the 1,6- linkages are resistant to amylase. As much as one third of amylopectin cannot be hydrolyzed by amylase. The average α-limit dextrin contains 5 to 10 glucose residues and is rapidly hydrolyzed by membrane bound enzymes.

FIGURE 11-3 ■ Products of starch hydrolysis by α-amylase.

Products of amylase action on starch and other major dietary sugars are hydrolyzed by brush border carbohydrases. The process (Figure 11-4) begins with the removal of α-limit dextrins. Glucoamylase is the most active enzyme, but sucrase and isomaltase also cleave these bonds. The glucose residues are removed sequentially from the nonreducing ends until a 1-6 branch point is reached. This bond is hydrolyzed by isomaltase, which also is called α-dextrinase. Sucrase cleaves 100% of sucrose to yield glucose and fructose. All lactose is broken down into glucose and galactose by lactase. Trehalase breaks the α-1,1- bonds of trehalose into glucose. Sucrase, lactase, and trehalose break down sucrose, lactose, and trehalose, respectively.

Sucrase and isomaltase occur together as a molecular complex. The fact that congenital deficiencies of sucrase and α-dextrinase occur together reveals a close functional relationship between these two enzymes. In humans sucrase-isomaltase is a compound molecule, one unit with absolute specificity for sucrose and one for the α-1,6- linkage of an α-limit dextrin.

In general there is a large disaccharidase reserve in the small intestine, so much that the rate-limiting step in sugar assimilation is not digestion but the absorption of free hexoses following hydrolysis. Under normal circumstances the major portion of sugar assimilation is complete in the proximal jejunum. The human GI tract does not possess cellulase capable of digesting the β-glucose bonds of cellulose and hemicellulose. These carbohydrates account for the undigestible fiber present in the diet.

Absorption of Digestion Products

For the body to utilize food-derived monosaccharides, they must be absorbed. Figure 11-5 shows how glucose absorption from the intestine occurs by passive as well as active processes. Although there are aqueous channels between enterocytes and pores in brush border membranes, dietary hexoses are too large to penetrate the membranes in any significant degree by passive diffusion. In humans the major routes of absorption are via three membrane carrier systems: SGLT-1, GLUT-5, and GLUT-2.

Fructose is transported by facilitated diffusion. The carrier involved is GLUT-5, which is located in the

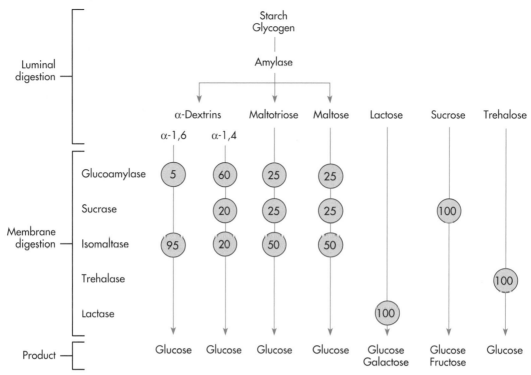

FIGURE 11-4 ■ Summary of carbohydrate digestion. *Circled numbers* denote the approximate percentage of substrate hydrolyzed by a particular brush border enzyme. The same carrier actively transports glucose and galactose into the cell, while fructose is absorbed by facilitated diffusion.

apical membrane of the enterocyte. The transport process does not depend on either Na^+ or energy. Fructose exits the basolateral membrane by another facilitated diffusion process involving the GLUT-2 transporter. GLUT-2 also is responsible for the exit of glucose and galactose from the absorbing cell.

The carrier systems for fructose and glucose and/or galactose differ insofar as the fructose carrier cannot be energized for active transport, whereas the glucose carrier can. Glucose and galactose are absorbed by secondary active transport via an Na^+-dependent carrier system (SGLT-1) (Figure 11-6). Mutual inhibition of glucose or galactose transport by the presence of the other indicates that they are transported by a common carrier.

The glucose entry step depicted in Figure 11-6 involves a carrier that binds sodium and galactose or glucose molecules; two Na^+ for each glucose or galactose molecule are transported into the cell. The entry step

is only slightly reversible because of removal of intracellular Na^+ by the pump on the basolateral membrane. Energy input (adenosine triphosphate [ATP]) drives the sodium pump and maintains a Na^+ gradient favoring glucose entry. Inhibition of the Na^+,K^+-ATPase with specific chemicals (such as ouabain) or interference of cellular energy production leads to cytosolic accumulation of Na^+ and the abolition of active sugar transport. The exit of glucose from the cytosol into the intracellular space is attributed partly to diffusion but mostly to facilitated diffusion via a Na^+-independent carrier located at the basolateral membrane; this carrier has specificity for all three hexoses (GLUT-2).

Regulation of Absorption

The capacity of the human small intestine to absorb free sugars is enormous. It has been estimated that hexoses equivalent to 22 pounds of sucrose can be

FIGURE 11-5 ■ Absorption rates of glucose from a solution perfused through the intestine of a guinea pig. In the absence of oxygen the rate of mediated uptake is proportional to concentration. When oxygen is available for cellular respiration the uptake is greater, and the carrier system can be energized for active transport. mM/L, millimoles/liter; μM/hr, micromoles/hour. *(Modified from Ricklis E, Quastel JH: Can J Biochem Physiol 36:348-362, 1958.)*

absorbed daily. There appears to be little physiologic control of sugar absorption. However, chemoreceptors and osmoreceptors in the proximal small intestine control the motility and emptying of the stomach through a negative feedback process mediated by hormones and neural reflexes. As an example, a volume of isotonic citrate solution of 750 milliliters (mL) placed in the human stomach passes into the small bowel in 20 minutes. The volume delivered in the same time is reduced if sucrose or glucose is added to the citrate solution. The amount delivered is related inversely to the sugar concentration.

Abnormalities in Carbohydrate Assimilation

It is obvious from the foregoing considerations that polysaccharides and oligosaccharides are absorbed as monosaccharides. Carbohydrates remaining in the intestinal lumen increase the osmotic pressure of the luminal contents because of defects in digestion and absorption. Bacterial fermentation of these carbohydrates in the lower small intestine and colon adds to this

osmotic effect. The osmotic retention of water in the lumen leads to diarrhea, bloating, and abdominal pain.

Diarrhea caused by the poor assimilation of dietary carbohydrates is most commonly caused by deficiencies in carbohydrate-splitting enzymes in the intestinal brush border. **Lactase deficiency,** the most frequently observed congenital disaccharidase deficiency, can exist in the absence of any other intestinal malfunction. The inability to digest lactose is actually a developmental change. In fact, a large percentage of the individuals of most races, other than those originating in Northern Europe, lose lactase activity later in life. Intolerance of sucrose and isomaltose is a rare disease found primarily in children. Intolerance of maltose has not been documented. The observation that lactase deficiency is a relatively common genetic disease, while maltase deficiency is not, may be related to the fact that only one enzyme displays significant lactase activity, whereas several display activity against maltose (see Figure 11-4). Thus maltose intolerance would require the simultaneous absence of all enzymes possessing maltase activity. Maldigestion of starch in humans is nonexistent because pancreatic amylase is secreted in tremendous excess.

Intolerance to glucose and galactose has been documented in rare instances. In these cases the patients thrive and show no symptoms when fed fructose. The explanation for this is found in the specificity of sugar absorption. Glucose and chemically related sugars are absorbed by a Na^+-dependent secondary active transport process, whereas fructose is absorbed by Na^+-independent facilitated diffusion. Thus, in these patients, the SGLT-1 transporter is absent, whereas GLUT-5 is present.

Besides defects in carbohydrate assimilation caused by the congenital or acquired enzyme deficiencies, assimilation of dietary sugars may be impaired by diseases of the GI tract. Celiac disease, certain bacterial infections, and some protozoan and helminth infections are associated with inflammation and structural derangements in the small bowel mucosa. These conditions are often attended by brush border enzyme deficiencies and hexose malabsorption (Figure 11-7). It is not uncommon to find lactase deficiency as a long-term consequence of intestinal disease, because this enzyme is present in the intestine at low levels compared with maltase and sucrase.

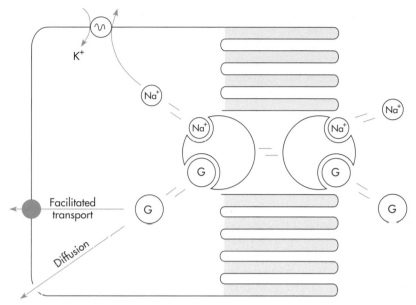

FIGURE 11-6 ■ Summary of a sodium-dependent carrier system for glucose-galactose (SGLT-1). Absorption involves the rapid movement from lumen to blood by an entry step and exit step mediated by two separate carrier molecules with specificity for hexose. The system is energized by an ATP-dependent Na⁺ pump that maintains a sodium gradient favoring the entry of 2 Na⁺ into the cell, with the concomitant cotransport of glucose or galactose (G). When Na⁺ is pumped from the cell, more Na⁺ and glucose are transported into the cell from the lumen. A carrier (GLUT-2) in the basolateral membrane facilitates the exit of fructose, as well as glucose and galactose, from the cell. The transport capacity of GLUT-2 appears to equal that involved in hexose entry, because hexose does not accumulate within the cells to a significant degree.

Symptoms of osmotic diarrhea include cramps and abdominal distention. An oral tolerance test can be used to diagnose disaccharidase deficiency if this is a suspected cause. After an overnight fast, adult patients are fed 50 g of lactose in a 10% aqueous solution (children are usually fed 2 g/kilogram [kg] of body weight). Blood samples are taken for glucose analysis before and at 5, 10, 15, 30, 45, and 60 minutes after lactose administration. An increase in blood glucose of at least 25 milligrams/deciliter (mg/dL) over fasted levels indicates normal hydrolysis of lactose and normal absorption of the glucose product. A flat lactose tolerance curve or failure to observe a rise in blood glucose over 25 mg/dL following lactose ingestion indicates low lactase activity. A value between 20 and 25 mg/dL is questionable. In this case the test may be repeated or, if laboratory facilities permit, intestinal biopsy specimens can be collected and examined for enzyme activity. In dealing with biopsy specimens, enzyme activity

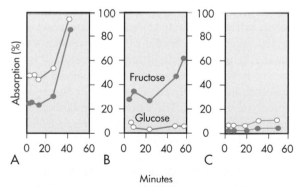

FIGURE 11-7 ■ Relative rates of absorption of fructose and glucose in an equimolar mixture studied by an intubation technique in a control subject (**A**), a patient with glucose malabsorption (**B**), and a patient with celiac disease (**C**). *(From Dahlquist A: In Sipple HL, McNutt KW (eds): Sugars in Nutrition. New York, Academic Press, 1974.)*

usually is expressed as units per gram of tissue protein. Tolerance tests for disaccharides other than lactose are seldom performed, but a similar procedure would suffice. Glucose or galactose tolerance tests should be performed to exclude monosaccharide malabsorption as the cause of a flat lactose tolerance curve.

PROTEIN ASSIMILATION

Digestion

Protein digestion begins in the stomach with the action of pepsin. The enzyme precursor pepsinogen is secreted by chief cells in response to a meal and low gastric pH. Acid in the stomach is responsible for activating pepsinogen to pepsin. Three pepsin isozymes have been recognized. All have a pH optimum of 1 to 3 and are denatured above pH 5. Pepsin is an endopeptidase with specificity for peptide bonds involving aromatic L-amino acids.

Pepsin activity terminates when the gastric contents mix with alkaline pancreatic juice in the small bowel. Chyme in the intestine stimulates the release of secretin and cholecystokinin (CCK), which in turn causes the pancreas to secrete bicarbonate and enzymes into the intestinal lumen.

There are two general classes of pancreatic proteases, **endopeptidases** and **exopeptidases.** The basis of classification and the particular characteristics of specific enzymes belonging to each class are given in Table 11-1.

Pancreatic proteases are secreted into the duodenum as inactive precursors. **Trypsinogen,** which lacks proteolytic activity, is activated by **enterokinase,** an enzyme located on the brush border of duodenal enterocytes. The exact chemical composition of enterokinase is not known; however, the fact that the molecule is 41% carbohydrate probably prevents its rapid digestion by proteolytic enzymes. The activity of enterokinase is stimulated by trypsinogen, and it is released from the brush border membrane by bile salts. Enterokinase activates trypsinogen by releasing a hexapeptide from the N-terminal end of the precursor molecule (Figure 11-8). Active trypsin, once formed, acts autocatalytically in the manner of enterokinase to activate the bulk of trypsinogen. Trypsin also activates other peptidase precursors from the pancreas (see Figure 11-8). **Chymotrypsinogen** is activated by cleavage of the peptide bond between arginine and isoleucine, which

TABLE 11-1	
Principal Pancreatic Proteases	
ENZYME	PRIMARY ACTION
Endopeptidases	Hydrolyze interior peptide bonds of polypeptides and proteins
Trypsin	Attacks peptide bonds involving basic amino acids; yields products with basic amino acids at C-terminal end
Chymotrypsin	Attacks peptide bonds involving aromatic amino acids, leucine, glutamine, and methionine; yields peptide products with these amino acids at C-terminal end
Elastase	Attacks peptide bonds involving neutral aliphatic amino acids; yields products with neutral amino acids at C-terminal end
Exopeptidases	Hydrolyze external peptide bonds of polypeptides and protein
Carboxypeptidase A	Attacks peptides with aromatic and neutral aliphatic amino acids at C-terminal end
Carboxypeptidase B	Attacks peptides with basic amino acids at C-terminal end

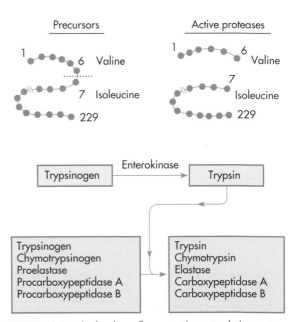

FIGURE 11-8 ■ Activation of pancreatic proteolytic enzymes. The process begins in the lumen when enterokinase cleaves a hexapeptide from trypsinogen, converting it to the active enzyme trypsin.

are the fifteenth and sixteenth amino acid residues at the N-terminus. Although structural rearrangement occurs, no peptide fragment is released because of a disulfide bond between the cysteine residues at positions 1 and 122 in the protein chain. This configuration is the active form of chymotrypsinogen. Cleavage at other points in the chymotrypsinogen molecule produces other molecular species of chymotrypsin having relatively little physiologic importance. The exact mechanism for activation of **proelastase** is not known, and activation of **procarboxypeptidases A and B** is relatively complicated, involving proteolysis of at least two proenzymes.

Once in the small intestine, pancreatic enzymes undergo rapid inactivation because of autodigestion. Trypsin is the enzyme primarily responsible for inactivation.

Development of Pancreatitis

In developed countries, 80% of the cases of acute pancreatitis are the result of either biliary stone disease or ethanol abuse. Alcohol consumption is the major cause of chronic pancreatitis.

As pointed out previously, trypsin plays a central role in the activation of other pancreatic zymogens. Normally trypsin remains as inactive trypsinogen until secreted into the duodenal lumen. The mechanisms responsible for the intracellular activation of trypsin are not totally clear. One hypothesis states that it is catalyzed by lysosomal hydrolases after the co-localization of these hydrolases with digestive zymogens within membrane-bound organelles during the early stages of pancreatitis.

Premature activation of trypsinogen within the pancreas initiates the entire activation cascade of other proteases, results in autodigestion of pancreatic cells, and causes acute pancreatitis. The body has a number of mechanisms to prevent premature trypsin activation. These include synthesis of pancreatic trypsin inhibitors, isolation of zymogens from lysosomes, and a site on trypsin that is susceptible to digestion by trypsin itself. Thus, when trypsin comes into contact with other trypsin molecules, it is able to cleave them and irreversibly inactivate the enzyme.

This site for autodigestion is an arginine residue in position 117. Recent research has located a single guanine-to-adenine gene mutation that results in histidine being substituted for arginine (R117H). This substitution prevents trypsin from being inactivated and was discovered in several families of patients with hereditary pancreatitis. Thus this mutation eliminates one of the failsafe mechanisms preventing the premature activation of trypsinogen and is the basis for at least one form of hereditary pancreatitis.

Absorption of Digestion Products

Membrane digestion and absorption are closely related phenomena in protein assimilation, and physiologists have been occupied by two fundamental questions concerning them: (1) In what form do products of proteolysis cross the brush border membrane of the epithelial cell? (2) In what form do these products leave the cell to enter the blood?

L-Isomers of some amino acids are absorbed by carrier-mediated mechanisms in much the same manner as glucose is absorbed. As with glucose, the cell entry process requires Na^+ as part of a ternary complex (see Figure 11-6), and uphill transfer occurs by secondary active transport. Other amino acids and some of those absorbed by active transport can also be absorbed by facilitated diffusion processes that do not require Na^+ (Table 11-2). A new class of electrogenic

TABLE 11-2		
Carrier Systems for the Transport of Amino Acids		
TRANSPORT SYSTEM	SUBSTRATE	DEPENDENCE ON Na^+ GRADIENT
Brush border membrane		
Neutral	All neutral aromatic and aliphatic AA	Yes
PHE	Phenylalanine and methionine	Yes
Acidic	Glutamate, aspartate	Yes
Imino	Proline, hydroxyproline	Yes
y^+	Basic AA	No
L	Neutral AA with hydrophobic side chains	No
Basolateral membrane		
A	Small neutral AA	Yes
ASC	Three- and four-carbon neutral AA	Yes
L	Neutral AA with hydrophobic side chains	No
y^+	Basic AA	No

AA, amino acids.

proton-dependent *a*mino acid *t*ransporters—PAT proteins—has been cloned. Present on the apical membrane, PAT proteins transport short-chain amino acids (glycine, alanine, serine, proline) into the cell, along with a hydrogen ion. Thus, the entry of the amino acid is coupled to the movement of a proton down its electrochemical gradient.

Certain L-amino acids compete with one another for uptake by intestinal cells. Studies of competition have led to the recognition of several different carrier systems for amino acid absorption (see Table 11-2). There is little doubt that the absorption of free amino acids by gut mucosa is physiologically important. However, amino acids appear in portal blood faster and reach a higher level when peptides from an acid hydrolysate of protein contact the gut mucosa than when there is an equimolar solution of free amino acid (Figure 11-9). Also, greater amounts of total nitrogen are absorbed from a solution of trypsin hydrolysate of proteins than from an equivalent solution of amino

acids in free form. Competition for transport between two chemically related amino acids is not observed when the same two acids are absorbed after ingestion of their dipeptides and tripeptides. In addition, the site in the intestine for the maximum absorption of amino acids in small peptide form is different from that for the absorption of free amino acids. The current explanation of these findings is that a separate carrier system for small peptides is involved in absorption. For example, free glycine absorption requires an amino acid carrier system. If saturation of the system occurs under physiologic conditions, the maximum rate of uptake becomes limiting. If, however, a second carrier for dipeptides or tripeptides of glycine is present, the amino acids can enter the cell in small-peptide form. Thus, two separate systems for glycine entry exist and work in a parallel manner.

The prevailing concepts regarding protein assimilation are illustrated in Figure 11-10. Luminal digestion of a protein meal produces approximately 40% free amino acids and 60% small peptides. As with the free acids, dipeptides and tripeptides resulting from digestion can be absorbed intact by a carrier-mediated process. However, tetrapeptides, pentapeptides, and hexapeptides are poorly absorbed; instead they are hydrolyzed by brush border peptidases to free amino acids or smaller absorbable peptides. Small peptides probably are absorbed by a single carrier with broad specificity. This is a secondary active transport process dependent on the Na+ gradient.

Peptides that enter enterocytes are hydrolyzed by cytoplasmic peptidases to amino acids. These, in turn, diffuse or are moved by carrier-mediated processes from the intracellular compartment, across the basolateral membrane, into the blood. As was the case with the apical membrane, a number of different carriers exist in the basolateral membrane (see Table 11-2). Some of these also are Na+-dependent. A small percentage of peptides enter the blood intact, which may explain why certain biologically active peptides exert their effects when given orally.

FIGURE 11-9 ■ Jejunal rates of glycine and leucine absorption (mean ± SEM, five subjects) from perfusion of test solutions containing either L-glycyl–L-leucine or an equimolar mixture of free L-glycine and free L-leucine. *(From Adibi SA: J Clin Invest 50:2266-2275, 1971.)*

Abnormalities in Protein Assimilation

Pancreatic insufficiency caused by various diseases, including cystic fibrosis and hereditary pancreatitis, may be associated with a decrease or absence of trypsin

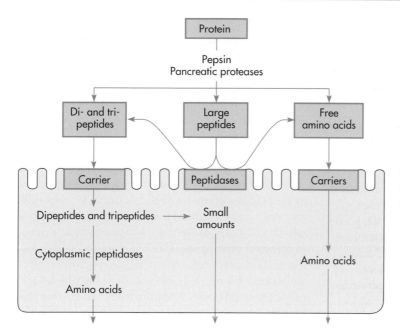

FIGURE 11-10 ■ Summary of the digestion and absorption of protein. Luminal digestion yields 40% free amino acids and 60% peptides consisting primarily of two to six amino acid residues.

and may lead to poor digestion of protein. Cases of primary proteinase deficiency caused by congenital trypsinogen deficiency have been reported. In those patients, chymotrypsin and carboxypeptidase activities are lacking also, because trypsin cannot be formed to activate the precursors of these pancreatic proteases.

Intestinal malabsorption of amino acids occurs in various hereditary diseases. Knowledge of intestinal transport abnormalities of this type is important not only for understanding the pathogenesis of certain diseases but also for providing important information regarding the physiologic process involved in intestinal transport.

Cystinuria is a disease characterized partly by defective transport of cystine in the proximal renal tubule and the small bowel (Figure 11-11). Although the intestinal malabsorptive condition is of little or no consequence in the disability produced by cystinuria, the fact that it is limited to the basic amino acids is supportive evidence that specific carrier systems exist for the intestinal uptake of amino acids.

Hartnup disease is a hereditary condition in which the active transport of several neutral amino acids is deficient in both the renal tubules and the small intestine. The intestinal defect contributes to the pathogenesis of

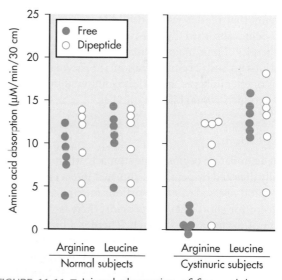

FIGURE 11-11 ■ Jejunal absorption of free arginine and leucine during perfusion of solutions containing L-arginine (1 mM) and L-leucine (1 mM) or L-arginyl–L-leucine (1 mM). Results are from studies carried out in six normal subjects and six cystinuric patients. *(From Silk DBA, Dawson AM. In Crane RK, Guyton AC (eds): International Review of Physiology. III: Gastrointestinal Physiology. Baltimore, University Park Press, 1979.)*

this disorder. An interesting finding is that, although neutral amino acids are not absorbed, they readily appear in the blood after ingestion of their dipeptides. This is compelling evidence that absorption of the dipeptides of certain amino acids is by a completely separate process from the one involved in the transport of free amino acids.

LIPID ASSIMILATION

Dietary lipids are complex organic compounds and include such substances as triacylglycerides (fat droplets), fat-soluble vitamins (A, D, E, and K), phospholipids, sterols, hydrocarbons, and waxes that compose cell walls or membranes of plants and/or animals. The principles of lipid assimilation are dealt with through a consideration of **triglycerides, phospholipids,** and **sterols.** The propensity of lipids to form ester linkages and the insolubility of lipids in water are important properties to keep in mind in relation to digestion and absorption.

Unlike carbohydrates and proteins, lipids enter epithelial cells by a sequence of chemical and physical events that render water-insoluble molecules capable of being absorbed by passive diffusion. The process depends on four major events: (1) secretion of bile and various lipases, (2) emulsification, (3) enzymatic hydrolysis of ester linkages, and (4) the solubilization of lipolytic products within bile salt micelles.

Digestion

Fat assimilation begins in the stomach, where food (partially digested by pepsin) is churned into a coarse mixture and released in small portions into the duodenum. Except for short-chain fatty acids, there is no absorption of fat from the stomach. There is a process, controlled through the action of CCK, that slows gastric motility and emptying when fat is in the small intestine. CCK also stimulates the pancreas to secrete lipase and causes contraction of the gallbladder. One function of bile salts released into the duodenum is to perpetuate the **emulsification** of fat droplets by decreasing the surface tension at the oil-water interface. An emulsification is a suspension of fat droplets held apart by phosphatidylcholine (lecithin), bile salts, fatty acids, and other emulsifying agents. The emulsified fat droplets

are approximately 1 micrometer (μm) in diameter. The emulsification process is important to increase the surface area of lipids in preparation for their enzymatic hydrolysis and is begun by the churning action of the stomach, which breaks contents into small droplets.

Enzymes from three sources are involved in the digestion of dietary lipids. These enzymes are food-bearing lipases, gastric lipase, and pancreatic lipases.

Enzymes that digest dietary lipids can be found in food per se (e.g., acid lipases, phospholipases). These enzymes may function in autodigestion, a process aided by the acid environment of the stomach. Human milk contains a lipase identical in chemical properties to bile salt–stimulated lipase secreted by the pancreas. Known as **carboxyl ester lipase** (CEL), it is active against cholesterol and vitamin A esters. CEL also hydrolyzes glycerol esters of long-chain fatty acids at the physiologic pH of the small bowel. A feature that distinguishes this esterase from well-known pancreatic lipase is that the latter has pronounced specificity for the 1 and 3 ester bonds of triglycerides, whereas CEL shows no positional specificity. Despite the lack of a clear functional role, it is presumed that CEL is important to the utilization of milk lipids in newborn infants, who have a low intestinal bile salt concentration and absorb glycerol and free fatty acids better than monoglycerides. This presumption is compatible with knowledge that CEL is stable between pH 3.5 and 9 and is broken down only slowly by pepsin. Thus, most of the enzyme would pass through the infant's stomach without denaturation. The fact that it requires bile salts for activation suggests that it is not functional until it reaches the small intestine.

Lipolytic activity in the human stomach is due primarily to **gastric lipase** secreted by cells of the corpus and fundus. This enzyme has an acidic pH optimum, ranging from 3 to 6. Gastric lipase acts primarily at the outer ester linkages, producing fatty acids and diglycerides. Pancreatic lipase is normally produced in great excess, and the absence of gastric lipase would not alter fat digestion. However, the contribution of gastric lipase can be significant in newborns and patients with pancreatic lipase deficiency or inactivation, such as might occur in Zollinger-Ellison syndrome because of the acid environment of the duodenum.

Pancreatic lipase-colipase, phospholipase A_2, and cholesterol esterase (nonspecific lipase) all function within the intestinal lumen.

Pancreatic lipase, or glycerol ester lipase, is secreted in an active form, rather than as a precursor enzyme. It displays optimum activity at pH 8, remains active down to pH 5, and is denatured at pH 3.5—irreversibly so at pH 2.5. Although bile salts inhibit its enzymatic activity, this is prevented under physiologic circumstances by the combination of lipase with **colipase.** Colipase, a polypeptide (102 to 107 amino acids) secreted by the pancreas along with lipase in a 1:1 ratio, is secreted as procolipase that is activated when hydrolyzed by trypsin to a peptide containing 96 amino acids. Whereas lipase-colipase complexes are scarce within the duodenum during fasting, the presence of fat stimulates the secretion of these components in large quantities. The inactivation of lipase by bile salts is due to the capacity of bile salts to displace lipase at the fat droplet–water interface, where it must exert its action. Colipase prevents inactivation by anchoring lipase to the oil-water interface in the presence of bile salts. Once colipase attaches to the fat droplet, lipase will bind to a specific site on the colipase molecule in a 1:1 ratio and consequently carry out its catalytic function, breaking down triglycerides. Colipase also has the capacity to bind to a bile salt micelle. Therefore, the products of fat hydrolysis need diffuse only a short distance to a micelle.

Lipase is secreted in large excess and rapidly hydrolyzes triglycerides. The enzyme shows positional specificity. It cleaves the 1 and 3 ester linkages, yielding free fatty acids and 2-monoglycerides. Only small amounts of free glycerol (Figure 11-12) are produced, reflecting the lack of action against the 2 ester linkages.

Phospholipase A₂ is secreted as a proenzyme and is activated by trypsin in much the same fashion as trypsinogen is converted to active form (i.e., through cleavage of several amino acids from the N-terminus). Bile salts and phospholipids form mixed micelles that become substrates for phospholipase A_2. The enzyme requires bile salts for optimal activity in hydrolyzing dietary phospholipids at the 2 position and producing lysophospholipid and free fatty acids.

Human pancreatic **cholesterol esterase** hydrolyzes not only cholesterol esters but also the esters of vitamins A, D, and E and those of glycerides. In contrast with pancreatic lipase, cholesterol esterase hydrolyzes all three ester linkages of triglycerides. This capacity accounts for its name—**nonspecific esterase.** Cholesterol esterase is active against substrates that have been incorporated into bile salt micelles. Activity is apparently dependent on the presence of specific bile salts. The enzyme in humans attacks cholesterol ester in the presence of taurocholate and taurochenodeoxycholate and is probably identical to CEL, which was previously discussed.

Absorption of Lipolytic Products

In addition to the function just mentioned, bile salts perform an important function in the actual absorption of lipolytic products. Sodium glycocholic and taurocholic acids, which are major bile salts, have both

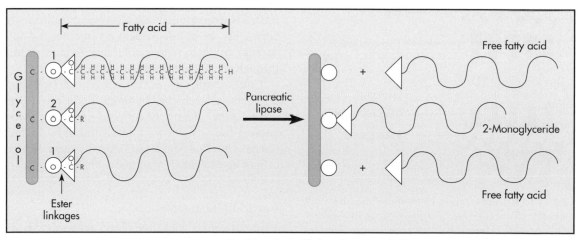

FIGURE 11-12 ■ Positional specificity of pancreatic lipase.

hydrophobic and hydrophilic portions. When their concentration in the intestine is raised to a critical level, bile salt monomers form water-soluble aggregates called **micelles.** The concentration of bile salt at which molecular aggregation occurs is referred to as the **critical micellar concentration.** Conjugated bile salts have a lower critical micellar concentration than unconjugated ones. Whereas emulsion particles are 2,000 to 50,000 angstroms (Å) in diameter, mixed micelles are about 30 to 100 Å in diameter, with a hydrophilic outer surface and a hydrophobic center. In addition, although emulsion particles form a suspension, micelles are in true solution. The water-insoluble monoglycerides from lipolysis are solubilized within the hydrophobic center of the micelle (Figure 11-13). In turn, fatty acids, lysophospholipids, cholesterol, and fat-soluble vitamins may be solubilized. A mixed micellar solution is water-clear. Micellar solubilization is important because it enhances the diffusion of poorly soluble dietary lipids through the unstirred aqueous layer overlying the enterocytes.

Two forms of evidence support the participation of micelles in the assimilation of fatty substances. First, mixed micelles (bile salts plus lipids) are found in the intestine. Second, long-chain fatty acids and monoglycerides are absorbed more rapidly from micellar solutions than from emulsions.

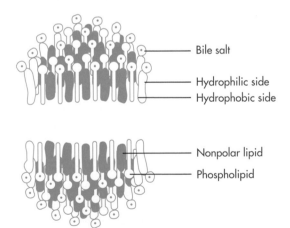

FIGURE 11-13 ■ Solubilization of nonpolar lipid by a bile acid–polar lipid micelle. *(Modified from Hoffman AF, French A, Littman A: Syllabus: Digestion and Absorption. Chicago, American Medical Association, 1975.)*

- Bile salt
- Hydrophilic side
- Hydrophobic side
- Nonpolar lipid
- Phospholipid

One possible mechanism of lipid uptake by enterocytes is the absorption of the entire mixed micelle. This proposed mechanism is not accepted, however, because various lipolytic products are absorbed at different rates. Also, because bile salts are absorbed in the ileum and lipid absorption usually is completed in the midjejunum, it is unlikely that the whole micelle enters the intestinal epithelium. Once bile salt absorption takes place, the bile salts are transported back to the liver for resecretion. The process of bile secretion, absorption, and return to the liver is referred to as the **enterohepatic circulation.**

The importance of micellar solubilization lies in the ability of micelles to diffuse across the unstirred water layer and present large amounts of fatty acids and monoglycerides to the apical membrane of the enterocyte. The brush border membrane is separated from the bulk solution in the intestinal lumen by the unstirred water layer. Single fatty acid and monoglyceride molecules, being poorly soluble in water, move slowly through this barrier. Because uptake depends on the number of molecules in contact with the enterocyte membrane, their absorption will be diffusion-limited. By contrast, micelles are water soluble, diffuse readily through the unstirred layer, and increase the concentration of fatty acids and monoglycerides at the membrane by 100- to 1000-fold. An acidic microclimate exists next to the plasma membrane, which protonates fatty acids, assisting in their release from the micelle and promoting their flux across the apical membrane. Thus, mixed micelles keep the intestinal water layer saturated with fatty acids, and absorption proceeds at an optimal rate. Short- and medium-chain fatty acids are not dependent on micelles for uptake because of their higher solubility in and diffusion through the unstirred aqueous layer.

Until recently, it was thought that all fat digestion products were absorbed by simple diffusion. However, there is now evidence of carrier-dependent processes. Some products such as linoleate show saturable uptake. Uptake in some cases exhibits a specificity that cannot be explained by simple diffusion.

Intracellular Events

Monoglycerides and free fatty acids absorbed by enterocytes are resynthesized into triglycerides by two diffcrcnt pathways: the major one, monoglyceride acylation, and the minor one, phosphatidic acid acylation (Figure 11-14).

Monoglyceride Acylation Pathway The monoglyceride acylation pathway involves the synthesis of triglycerides from 2-monoglycerides and coenzyme A (CoA)–activated fatty acids. Acyl-CoA synthetase is the enzyme that acylates fatty acids. The enzymes monoglyceride and diglyceride acyltransferases are responsible for catalyzing the formation of diglycerides and

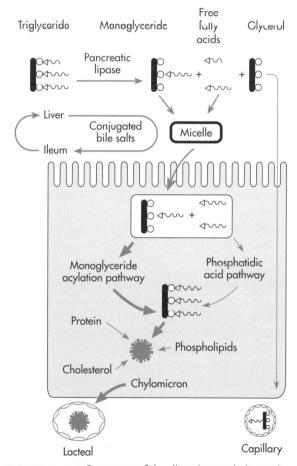

FIGURE 11-14 ■ Summary of the digestion and absorption of triglyceride. Monoglycerides and long-chain fatty acids enter the cells after first being incorporated into micelles. Glycerol and short- and medium-chain acids, because of their solubility in the aqueous unstirred layer, enter without micelle solubilization.

triglycerides, respectively. The enzymes involved in this pathway are associated mainly with the smooth endoplasmic reticulum.

An interesting aspect of intracellular triglyceride synthesis is that certain fatty acids are used in preference to others. This occurs despite similar rates of absorption by enterocytes and similar rates of enzymatic CoA activation and glyceride esterification. These observations have been explained by the presence of intracellular **fatty acid–binding proteins** (FABPs), which have affinities for fatty acids of different chain lengths and varying degrees of saturation. Such proteins exert their influence after absorption occurs and before esterification takes place.

A current theory on how FABPs operate presumes that absorbed fatty acids bind strongly to the apical membrane of enterocytes. Solubilization is brought about when the fatty acids bind specifically with receptors on FABPs. This facilitates the transfer of the free fatty acids from the apical membrane to the smooth endoplasmic reticulum, where esterification into diglycerides and triglycerides takes place. This process is particularly effective in the intracellular transfer of long-chain fatty acids. By binding fatty acids, FABPs protect the cell from high concentrations of fatty acids that would be capable of solubilizing lipid membranes. Such a situation might occur during the digestion of a lipid meal. Short- and medium-chain fatty acids, which show less affinity for the cell membrane, are water soluble and not bound by specific proteins. Instead they leave the cell in free form and enter the blood directly, rather than as reesterified triglyceride in chylomicrons.

Phosphatidic Acid Pathway Triglycerides also can be synthesized from CoA-activated fatty acids and α-glycerophosphate. The latter is formed from phosphorylated glycerol or from the reduction of dihydroxyacetone phosphate derived from glycolysis. One mol of α-glycerophosphate acylated with 2 mol of CoA–fatty acids yields phosphatidic acid, which is dephosphorylated to form diglyceride, which in turn is acylated to form triglyceride. This minor pathway for triglyceride synthesis in the intestine is termed the *phosphatidic acid pathway*.

Phosphatidic acid may also be important in the synthesis of phospholipids such as phosphatidyl choline, ethanolamine, and serine. Alternatively, phospholipids can be derived from acylation of absorbed lysophospholipids by appropriate acyltransferases. The acylation of lysophosphatidyl choline forms phosphatidyl choline, which is used in the formation of chylomicrons.

Dietary cholesterol is absorbed in free form. However, a major fraction leaves the epithelial cells in chylomicrons as esters of fatty acids. This is indicative of the highly active intracellular reesterification process. The ratio of free to esterified cholesterol in intestinal lymph is influenced by the amount of cholesterol in the diet (low dietary cholesterol favors the cellular exit of greater amounts of free sterol in chylomicrons). In humans the percentage of net cholesterol absorption decreases as the dietary content increases.

Chylomicrons are lipoprotein particles about 750 to 5000 Å in diameter that are synthesized within enterocytes and exist in the form of an emulsion. Although their chemical composition may vary slightly depending on size, chylomicrons are approximately 80% to 90% triglycerides, 8% to 9% phospholipids, 2% cholesterol, 2% protein, and traces of carbohydrate. Recent studies suggest how triglycerides and esterified cholesterol and fat-soluble vitamins (which form the core) become coated with **apolipoprotein,** phospholipid, and free cholesterol (which make up the surface of the chylomicron). Synthesis of the chylomicron appears to be a two-step process. Small particles containing apolipoprotein B and a small mass of core lipids are synthesized in the rough endoplasmic reticulum. Microsomal triglyceride transfer protein (MTP) is responsible for adding lipids to apolipoprotein B. Concurrently, triglyceride-rich particles that lack apolipoprotein B are synthesized in the lumen of the smooth endoplasmic reticulum. The two particles join, forming a nascent chylomicron. This complex, in turn, is transported to the Golgi apparatus, where the apolipoprotein is glycosylated. The newly formed chylomicrons are secreted by exocytosis into the interstitial space and enter the gaps between the endothelial cells that make up the lacteals. Chylomicrons are too large to enter the pores of blood capillaries.

It is evident that apolipoprotein synthesis by epithelial cells and its incorporation into chylomicrons are essential for fat absorption. Inhibition of protein synthesis causes large amounts of triglyceride to accumulate intracellularly. Several apolipoproteins—termed A, B, C, and E—have been identified in intestinal lymph. Apolipoprotein B is similar immunologically to plasma very-low-density lipoprotein (VLDL) and low-density lipoprotein (LDL) but chemically and physically shows some uniqueness. It has been suggested that VLDL in plasma may represent chylomicrons of varying densities. The role of apolipoproteins in fat absorption and metabolism remains an area of active investigation.

Abnormalities in Lipid Assimilation

Impaired lipid assimilation is considered under the general title of malabsorption. In most cases all nutrients are malabsorbed to some extent. However, the clinical entity is defined in terms of fat malabsorption because, unlike carbohydrates and proteins, fat not absorbed in the small intestine passes through the colon and appears in the feces in a measurable form.

Presence of excessive fat in the stool can be established by extracting fecal samples with organic solvents and determining the total fatty acids present, excluding volatile short-chain acids. Less than 7 g of fecal fatty acid per day is normal. Values above this level suggest malabsorption or the carcinoid syndrome.

A convenient way to consider fat malabsorption is to review the various steps in assimilation and consider possible derangements in each. For each derangement, at least one possible disease has been recognized:

- Disorders of gastric mixing and intestinal motility do not have any clear-cut disease associated with them, although malabsorption may follow the rapid gastric emptying that accompanies partial gastrectomy. Also, rapid intestinal transit has been suggested as the basis for diarrhea in hyperthyroidism.
- Luminal digestion of triglycerides may be deranged by defects in pancreatic enzyme secretion or action. A quantitative defect would be caused by impaired enzyme synthesis and secretion, as occurs with cystic fibrosis (a congenital disease of exocrine glands) or chronic pancreatitis. It should be noted that normal digestion can proceed with as little as 5% to 10% of normal enzyme secretion. A qualitative defect would occur if the conditions for enzyme action were not optimal (as in gastric acid hypersecretion [Zollinger-Ellison syndrome], when the pH of the duodenal contents is lowered and lipase cannot function or

may even be denatured). A defect in pancreatic lipase results in the presence of triglycerides in the stool.

- Transport from the lumen is a special step in fat absorption and is dependent on a suitable bile acid concentration, which may be low because of a quantitative bile acid deficiency that occurs with an interrupted enterohepatic circulation (e.g., ileal resection or dysfunction, biliary obstruction or cholestatic liver disease). There may be a qualitative deficit of the bile acids in a condition known as the *bacterial overgrowth syndrome* (in which stasis in the upper intestine leads to bacterial overgrowth, with deconjugation of bile acids by the bacteria). Free bile acids are absorbed passively in the jejunum because they are largely un-ionized at the duodenal pH. Bile acids need to be ionized to form micelles. Therefore the un-ionized state leads to impairment of fat absorption as well as impaired absorption of cholesterol and fat-soluble vitamins. Bile acid deficiency does not interfere with digestion, so in this case free fatty acids and monoglycerides appear in the stool.

- Mucosal cell transport is, of course, necessary for all nutrients, but it is of particular importance in fat absorption, because the absorbed fatty acids or monoglycerides must be reconstituted to triglycerides and then formed into chylomicrons. No disease has been associated with triglyceride synthesis; however, there is a disease of inadequate chylomicron formation called *abetalipoproteinemia*. This condition is caused by a failure to synthesize MTP, which is necessary for the initial steps that bring apolipoprotein B together with triglyceride in the process of chylomicron formation. The synthesis of apolipoprotein B is in fact normal in affected persons—so the condition is misnamed.

- Lymphatic transport is necessary for the absorption of fat that has been reconstituted to chylomicrons. This step is defective in two rare diseases, congenital lymphangiectasia and Whipple's disease.

Thus, by considering the steps in fat absorption, it is possible to predict the diseases that can lead to malabsorption. Steatorrhea, which attends malabsorption, can be alleviated to a large degree by diets containing triglycerides of medium- rather than long-chain fatty acids. The explanation for the benefit of this dietary maneuver is that glycerol esters of medium-chain fatty acids are hydrolyzed faster than are ester linkages involving long-chain fatty acids. Medium-chain fatty acids are water soluble and can be absorbed from aqueous solution. Also, they are transported directly into portal blood without involvement of chylomicrons.

VITAMINS

Vitamins are organic compounds that cannot be manufactured by the body but are vital for metabolism. They are considered (in this instance) not on the basis of any physiologic function, but rather on the basis of whether they are water-soluble or fat-soluble (Table 11-3). This feature is emphasized because their solubility dictates the general mechanism by which vitamins are absorbed.

Water-soluble vitamins are represented by an array of compounds. The principles that apply to the absorption of hexoses and amino acids apply to the absorption of vitamins as well. Strongly ionized or high-molecular-weight compounds are absorbed poorly compared with non-ionized, low-molecular-weight substances.

Relatively little information exists regarding the processes involved in the intestinal uptake of vitamins. Most evidence suggests that passive diffusion is the predominant mechanism. Exceptions exist for thiamine, vitamin C, folic acid, and vitamin B_{12}, for which special transport mechanisms have been reported.

TABLE 11-3		
Solubility of Vitamins		
VITAMIN	FAT SOLUBLE	WATER SOLUBLE
A	+	
B_1 (thiamine)		+
B_2 (riboflavin)		+
Niacin		+
C (ascorbic acid)		+
D	+	
E	+	
K	+	
Folic acid		+
B_6 (pyridoxine, pyridoxal, pyridoxamine)		+
B_{12}		+
Pantothenic acid		+
Biotin		+

At low luminal concentrations, thiamine (vitamin B_1) can be absorbed in the jejunum of some species, including humans, by a Na^+-dependent, active process, whereas at high concentrations, passive diffusion predominates. The presence of a carrier-mediated transport system is suggested by the fact that metabolic inhibitors, thiamine analogues, and the absence of sodium all depress thiamine uptake by enterocytes. Riboflavin (vitamin B_2) is absorbed in the proximal small bowel by facilitated transport. Pyridoxine (vitamin B_6) is absorbed by simple diffusion.

Vitamin C is required in only a few species, including humans. Humans are capable of absorbing it from the intestine by passive processes and also by active transport (an energy-dependent process, requiring Na^+). In rats and hamsters, species that do not require ascorbic acid, uptake of the vitamin occurs only by passive mechanisms.

Folic acid has been reported as being transported actively in the duodenum and jejunum of humans and from the entire small intestine of some rodents. A mediated process might be predicted from two facts: folic acid is a strongly electronegative compound (with a molecular weight of 441), and uncouplers of respiration (hence, energy production) interfere with its absorption.

Vitamin B_{12} (cobalamin) absorption requires intrinsic factor, a glycoprotein secreted by the parietal cell of the gastric mucosa. Binding of intrinsic factor to dietary vitamin B_{12} is necessary for attachment to specific receptors located in the brush border of the ileum. Initially cobalamin is released from foods by the action of pepsin. Because of a higher affinity for R proteins (glycoproteins), which are secreted in gastric juice along with intrinsic factor, the vitamin and R proteins form a complex. When the R protein becomes digested in the duodenum, the vitamin then forms a complex with intrinsic factor that is resistant to digestion. The presence of Ca^{++} or Mg^{++} and an alkaline pH are necessary for optimal attachment of the intrinsic factor–B_{12} complex to the receptor, a process that does not require energy. The actual uptake of B_{12} is presumed to be by pinocytosis; however, this point is not clear. Any disease condition that interferes with the production or secretion of intrinsic factor or with the attachment of the intrinsic factor–B_{12} complex to its receptor in the ileum leads to malabsorption of vitamin B_{12}.

The fat-soluble vitamins (A, D, E, and K) depend on solubilization within bile salt micelles for intestinal absorption. Vitamin A, or retinol, is ingested as β-carotene and absorbed as such. Once in the enterocyte, β-carotene is cleaved intracellularly into two retinol molecules. Esters of dietary vitamins D and E, as noted earlier in this chapter, are digested by cholesterol ester hydrolase before their solubilization in micelles. Dietary vitamin K (K_1) is absorbed in the intestine by an active transport system, whereas bacterially derived K_2 is taken up passively from the lumen. Except for retinol, which is re-esterified, the fat-soluble vitamins appear in exocytosed chylomicrons biochemically unaltered by metabolic processes within the enterocyte. The chylomicrons are then extruded into the lymphatics and transported via the thoracic duct into the blood. Thus the absorption of fat-soluble vitamins depends on the absorption of dietary lipids. In fact, a fatty meal is necessary for absorption of reasonable amounts of vitamin E. Defects leading to fat malabsorption result in deficiencies of fat-soluble vitamins.

SUMMARY

1. Digestion is the chemical breakdown of food by enzymes secreted into the lumen of the gut and those associated with the brush border of enterocytes.
2. All physiologically significant absorption of nutrients occurs in the small intestine, the mucosal surface of which is greatly increased, providing a large area for uptake.
3. The major luminal breakdown of carbohydrates is catalyzed by amylase. Breakdown of remaining glucose polymers and other disaccharides is carried out by specific enzymes in the brush border membrane. Glucose and galactose share an Na^+-dependent, secondary active transport mechanism for absorption.
4. The major enzymes involved in the luminal digestion of protein are secreted in inactive forms by the

pancreas and then activated by trypsin following its own activation by enterokinase.

5. Dipeptides, tripeptides, and amino acids are absorbed across the brush border membrane by a variety of transport processes. Larger peptides are broken down into these absorbable forms by peptidases associated with the brush border. Absorbed small peptides are hydrolyzed to amino acids within the cytoplasm, and almost all absorbed protein leaves the enterocyte in the form of amino acids.

6. Fat droplets are suspended in an emulsification by the action of lecithin, bile salts, peptides, and other such agents. Colipase displaces a bile salt molecule from the fat-water interface, allowing pancreatic lipase to digest the triglycerides. Pancreatic lipase is essential to fat digestion and produces 2-monoglycerides and free fatty acids.

7. The breakdown products of fat digestion are solubilized in micelles by bile salts and other amphipathic molecules. Micelles diffuse through the unstirred layer, and fat digestion products are absorbed from the micelles at the enterocyte brush border membrane.

8. Within the enterocyte, triglycerides and phospholipids are resynthesized and packaged into chylomicrons that contain apoprotein on their surface. Chylomicrons are exocytosed into the intercellular space. Too large to enter capillaries, the chylomicrons enter lacteals and eventually reach the blood via the thoracic lymph duct.

KEY WORDS AND CONCEPTS

- Brush border
- Enterocytes
- Goblet cells
- Digestion
- Luminal/cavital digestion
- Contact/membrane digestion
- Unstirred layer of fluid
- Glycocalyx
- Passive diffusion
- Facilitated diffusion
- Active transport
- Starch
- Sucrose
- Lactose
- Maltose
- Amylopectin
- Lactase deficiency
- Endopeptidases
- Exopeptidases
- Trypsinogen
- Enterokinase
- Chymotrypsinogen
- Proelastase
- Procarboxypeptidases A and B
- Triglycerides
- Phospholipids
- Sterols
- Emulsification
- Carboxyl ester lipase
- Gastric lipase
- Pancreatic lipase
- Colipase
- Phospholipase A_2
- Cholesterol esterase
- Nonspecific esterase
- Micelles
- Critical micellar concentration
- Enterohepatic circulation
- Fatty acid–binding proteins
- Chylomicrons
- Apolipoprotein

REFERENCES

Ahnen DJ: Nutrient assimilation. In Kelly WN (ed): Textbook of Internal Medicine. Philadelphia, JB Lippincott, 1989.

Alpers DH: Digestion and absorption of carbohydrates and proteins. In Johnson LR (ed): Physiology of the Gastrointestinal Tract, 3rd ed. New York, Raven Press, 1994.

Ganapathy V, Ganapathy ME, Leibach FH: Intestinal transport of peptides and amino acids. Curr Top Med 50:379-412, 2001.

Hamilton RL, Wong JS, Cham CM, et al: Chylomicron-sized lipid particles are formed in the setting of apolipoprotein B deficiency. J Lipid Res 39:1543-1557, 1998.

Milne MD: Hereditary disorders of intestinal transport. In Smythe DH (ed): Intestinal Absorption. New York, Plenum Press, 1974.

Rose RC: Intestinal absorption of water-soluble vitamins. In Johnson LR (ed): Physiology of the Gastrointestinal Tract, 2nd ed. New York, Raven Press, 1987.

Solomon T: Pancreatic exocrine function. In Kelly WN (ed): Textbook of Internal Medicine. Philadelphia, JB Lippincott, 1989.

Tso P: Intestinal lipid absorption. In Johnson LR (ed): Physiology of the Gastrointestinal Tract, 3rd ed. New York, Raven Press, 1994.

Wellner D, Meister A: A survey of inborn errors of amino acid metabolism and transport in man. Annu Rev Biochem 50: 911-968, 1980.

Whitcomb DC: Hereditary pancreatitis: New insights into acute and chronic pancreatitis. Gut 45:317-322, 1999.

Wright EM, Hirayama BA, Loo DDF, et al: Intestinal sugar transport. In Johnson LR (ed): Physiology of the Gastrointestinal Tract, 3rd ed. New York, Raven Press, 1994.

12

FLUID AND ELECTROLYTE ABSORPTION

LEONARD R. JOHNSON

Minerals and water enter the body through the intestine and provide the solutes and solvent water for body fluids. The electrolytes of primary importance include Na^+, K^+, Cl^-, Ca^{++}, and Fe^{++}. Each of these ions has one or more mechanisms by which it is transported across the intestinal epithelium. This chapter considers these mechanisms and their relationship to water absorption and secretion.

BIDIRECTIONAL FLUID FLUX

During a 24-hour period, 7 to 10 liters (L) of water enters the small intestine (Figure 12-1). Fluid derived from food and drink accounts for approximately 2 L. The other 7 L is derived from the secretions of the gastrointestinal (GI) tract: saliva, 1 L; gastric juice, 2 L; pancreatic juice, 2 L; bile, 1 L; and small intestinal secretions, 1 L. Of the amount entering, only about 600 milliliters (mL) per 24-hour period reaches the colon, indicating that most water is absorbed in the small intestine. Because the average daily fecal weight is about 150 grams (g), of which 100 g is water, 500 mL of fluid is absorbed daily from the colon. This volume represents 10% to 25% of the absorptive capacity of the colon, which is capable of absorbing about 4 to 6 L of fluid per day. Malabsorption of solutes and water in the small intestine may result in enough fluid entering the colon to overwhelm its absorptive capacity and cause diarrhea. This, in turn, can precipitate severe electrolyte deficiencies. Although it is possible that ions and water may be added to the feces from colonic mucosa, the major source of water and electrolytes in a diarrheic stool is the small intestine (see Figure 12-1).

It is evident from the foregoing account that several liters of fluid are secreted into the GI tract daily, and several liters are absorbed. The volume of fluid moving from blood to lumen (secretion) is less than that moving from the lumen to the blood (absorption), resulting in net absorption. Absorption generally results from the passive movement of water across the epithelial membrane in response to osmotic and hydrostatic pressures. Because of these so-called *Starling forces*, the consequent bulk flow of fluid is analogous to the flow of fluid across capillary walls. In the absence of food, ions are the most important contributors to osmotic pressure in the intestinal lumen. The ionic composition of the luminal contents may vary along the length of the intestine and is different from that in feces. Luminal fluid generally remains isotonic with plasma, however, because of the relative permeability of the mucosal membrane. The continued production of solutes by colonic bacteria, together with the relative impermeability of the colonic membrane to water, usually causes stool water to be hypertonic, 350 to 400 milliosmoles (mOsm)/L, to plasma.

IONIC CONTENT OF LUMINAL FLUID

Osmotic equilibration with plasma of material entering the small bowel occurs rapidly in the duodenum. Water is absorbed from hypotonic solutions and enters

FIGURE 12-1 ■ Volume and composition of fluid in the small intestine and colon.

K+ concentration increases to 90 mEq/L, up from 9 mEq/L in the ileum. The major anions in the colon are Cl⁻ and HCO_3^-.

These values indicate an effective absorption process for Na+ that becomes increasingly efficient toward the distal portions of the gut. This is caused in part by a decrease in the permeability of the epithelium, preventing the back-diffusion of ions absorbed in the distal portions. Whereas the absorption of Na+ in the distal gut is effective, the conservation of Cl⁻ is even more so. Chloride is exchanged for metabolically derived HCO_3^-.

Potassium is absorbed passively by the small intestine as the volume of intestinal contents decreases. The concentration of K+ remains roughly equal to that in the serum (4 or 5 mEq/L). In the colon, net K+ secretion occurs. Because of K+ secretion and the exchange of Cl⁻ for HCO_3^- in the colon, prolonged diarrhea results in a hypokalemic metabolic acidosis.

TRANSPORT ROUTES AND PROCESSES

Ions move between the gut lumen and the blood through **transcellular** and **paracellular pathways.** The passive movement of Na+, both into and out of the lumen, is largely through the lateral spaces. This movement is regulated by the **tight junctions** or **zonulae occludens**. The rate of this passive component is affected by electrochemical gradients and Starling forces. Normally these forces are small and account for only a small fraction of the net transport. They can, however, be altered under certain conditions, with marked effects.

The tight junction is about twice as permeable to Na+ and K+ as it is to Cl⁻. Thus, electrical potentials can arise across this structure. If, for example, NaCl is moving across the tight junction, the Cl⁻ will be retarded relative to the Na+, and the surface toward which the movement is occurring will become positive relative to the other surface. Ions slightly larger than Na+ and K+ are much more restricted in their movement.

The pores through which transcellular diffusion takes place are probably larger (7 to 8 angstroms [Å]) in the proximal bowel than in the ileum (3 to 4 Å). This restricts the passive transport of solutes in distal gut and allows these solutes to exert a more effective osmotic pressure. In turn, the reduced permeability makes

hypertonic solutions. Na+ and Cl⁻ also leave hypertonic solutions. Most of this movement occurs through the relatively permeable junctions between the epithelial cells of the proximal small intestine.

Proceeding from the duodenum to the colon, the Na+ and Cl⁻ concentrations in the lumen progressively become lower than the plasma concentrations. In the duodenum, Na+ is approximately 140 mEq/L, equal to the serum concentration. The major anion is Cl⁻. Sodium concentrations decrease in the jejunum and reach about 125 mEq/L in the ileum. The major anions in the ileum are Cl⁻ and HCO_3^-. Sodium decreases to 35 to 40 mEq/L in the colon, whereas the carrier-mediated transport a more important contributor to net transport out of the lumen.

Na$^+$-Cl$^-$ Transport

Physiologic models describing Na$^+$ and Cl$^-$ absorption in the small intestine are shown in Figure 12-2. Sodium is absorbed from the lumen across the apical membrane of epithelial cells by four mechanisms. These include the movement of Na$^+$ by restricted diffusion through water-filled channels, the cotransport of Na$^+$ with organic solutes (e.g., glucose and amino acids), the cotransport of Na$^+$ with Cl$^-$, and the countertransport of Na$^+$ in exchange for H$^+$. Because Na$^+$-Cl$^-$ cotransport and Na$^+$-H$^+$ exchange are electrically neutral processes, the driving force for Na$^+$ to enter the cell is the Na$^+$ concentration difference between the luminal fluid and the cytoplasm. Sodium movement through pores and Na$^+$ cotransport with organic solutes are also driven by the Na$^+$ concentration difference but are electrogenic and increase the negative electrical potential across the epithelial cell membrane. The contribution of restricted diffusion to overall Na$^+$ absorption is probably small relative to other mechanisms.

The presence of these various mechanisms varies over the length of the small intestine. In the proximal bowel Na$^+$ is absorbed primarily coupled to H$^+$ countertransport and solute (amino acids and sugars) cotransport. In the ileum Na$^+$ is absorbed coupled to the absorption of Cl$^-$. Throughout the gut Cl$^-$ is absorbed along the electrical gradient. In the ileum, coupled Na$^+$ transport is the major carrier-mediated pathway for Cl$^-$ absorption. Exchange of Cl$^-$ for HCO$_3^-$ occurs in the distal ileum and increases dramatically in the colon and rectum. This mechanism accounts for the high HCO$_3^-$ content and alkaline pH of stool water.

The Na$^+$-K$^+$ pump on the basolateral membranes of the absorbing epithelial cell maintains both the low intracellular Na$^+$ level and the negative membrane potential. Through this pump the Na$^+$ that enters by all four mechanisms described previously is extruded into the intercellular spaces. The Na$^+$ pump is the well-known Na$^+$,K$^+$-activated adenosine triphosphatase (ATPase). This enzyme-carrier molecule is activated by intracellular Na$^+$ and extracellular K$^+$ to split ATP, releasing energy. In the process, three Na$^+$ ions are pumped out of the cell for every two K$^+$ ions pumped in. The pumping out of more Na$^+$ than there is K$^+$ entering creates a potential difference across the basolateral membrane, which is called an **electrogenic potential**. The pump is inhibited by cardiac glycosides (e.g., ouabain). Because Na$^+$ exit from the epithelial

FIGURE 12-2 ■ Mechanism of NaCl absorption in the small intestine. Sodium enters passively, following the electrochemical gradient, by cotransport with nutrients such as glucose or amino acids, or by neutral cotransport with Cl$^-$ or in exchange for protons via a countertransport process. Chloride also is absorbed by neutral exchange with HCO$_3^-$. Sodium exit from the cell is via the energy-dependent Na$^+$ pump, and Cl$^-$ follows passively. The electrical potential difference across the apical membrane is −40 mV, and across the entire cell is +3 to +5 mV with reference to the luminal side. Ouabain is an inhibitor of Na$^+$,K$^+$-ATPase. H$_2$CO$_3^-$, carbonic acid.

cell is coupled with K^+ entry, the intracellular K^+ concentration is much higher than the extracellular concentration. This causes the constant, downhill leakage of K^+ from the interior to the exterior by potassium channels on the basolateral membranes (i.e., the K^+ actively pumped into the cell returns to the exterior through passive leaks).

The epithelial absorption of Cl^- involves, in addition to cotransport with Na^+, countertransport with HCO_3^- (see Figure 12-2). Production of HCO_3^- is through a metabolic process taking place within the epithelial cells through the hydration of CO_2 by carbonic anhydrase. Both absorptive mechanisms move Cl^- into the epithelial cell against an electrochemical potential difference (PD). The energy for the uphill movement of Cl^- is derived from the downhill movement of Na^+ into the cell or from the downhill movement of HCO_3^- out of the cell and into the lumen.

Because of the transcellular electrical PD—the serosal side is positive with reference to the lumen and with reference to the cell interior—Cl^- is driven passively from the cell and into the serosal fluid. Also, luminal Cl^- can move through the paracellular pathway into the serosal solution. The magnitude of this passive absorptive process is governed by the magnitude of the transmural PD. That PD is developed through the action of the Na^+-K^+ pump and the absorption of Na^+ coupled to organic solutes. It is influenced by the resistance of the paracellular pathway to ion flow. In the small intestine the relatively leaky epithelium prevents the transmural PD from rising above 2 to 5 millivolts (mV). In the colon, where the epithelium is less leaky, the PD is about 20 mV. Thus the driving force for Cl^- absorption is greater in the colon.

All regions of the colon absorb Na^+ and Cl^- (Figure 12-3). Unlike in the small intestine, however, the cotransport of Na^+ with organic solutes is lacking. Restricted diffusion is the primary mechanism for colonic Na^+ absorption. This electrogenic process, which increases in activity from oral to aboral regions, is dependent on channels that are under regulation by mineralocorticoids. For example, aldosterone increases the number of sodium channels and enhances Na^+ absorption. Sodium in the lumen of the colon also is absorbed through an electroneutral process that includes Cl^- cotransport. This probably involves Na^+-H^+ countertransport coupled with Cl^--HCO_3^- countertransport, as occurs in the small intestine.

FIGURE 12-3 ■ Mechanism of ion absorption in the colon. Na^+ enters passively, whereas Cl^- enters in neutral exchange with HCO_3^-. Net secretion of K^+ occurs.

K⁺ Transport

Diffusion through paracellular pathways in the small intestine is the primary mechanism by which K^+, derived from the diet or from secretions of the upper GI tract, undergoes net absorption. In the colon (but not in the small intestine) the apical and basolateral membranes are permeable to K^+. Thus, because of the high concentration of intracellular K^+ maintained by the Na^+-K^+ pump, some K^+ leaks passively across the apical membrane of epithelial cells. Factors that elevate intracellular K^+, such as aldosterone-stimulated Na^+ absorption, increase K^+ secretion.

MECHANISM FOR WATER ABSORPTION AND SECRETION

Water absorption or secretion always occurs in response to osmotic forces produced by the transport of organic solutes or ions and can be explained in terms of a three-compartment model and local osmotic effects (Figure 12-4). In the absorbing intestine, solutes are moved from the lumen (first compartment) into and then out of the epithelial cell. This creates a local osmotic gradient, causing water to move from the gut lumen, across the cell, and into the intercellular space (second compartment). The entrance of water increases the hydrostatic pressure within this space, causing the bulk flow of water and solutes through the basement membrane into capillaries (third compartment). In the nonabsorbing intestine the imbalance of forces across the capillary wall leads to filtration of fluid into the interstitium. However, the capillary filtration rate is balanced by lymphatic drainage. In the secreting intestine, fluid in the interstitium is attracted osmotically into the lumen.

Osmotic equilibration, and thus absorption, occur by different means in the duodenum and the ileum. The duodenum functions to bring chyme into osmotic equilibrium with plasma. If a hypertonic solution is placed in the duodenum, isotonicity is reached by a rapid flow of water from blood to lumen, increasing the volume of the original solution. More distally, in the small intestine, absorption of solutes creates a gradient for water absorption. Thus the volume is decreased because of both solute and water uptake, and the isotonicity of the luminal solution is maintained

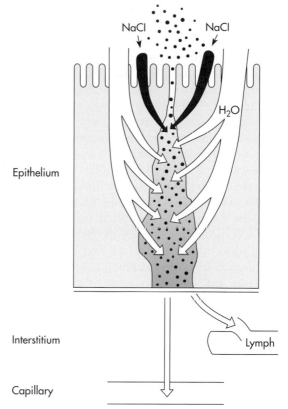

FIGURE 12-4 ■ Fluid absorption according to the standing osmotic gradient hypothesis. The sum of hydrostatic and osmotic pressures in the intraepithelial space, interstitium, and capillaries favors fluid absorption. In the nonabsorbing state, fluid filtering from the capillaries would be drained by the lymphatics. The attraction of fluid from the cytosol and interstitium due to high osmotic pressure in the lumen leads to secretion.

during this process. In summary, the sequence of responses to hypertonic contents entering the intestinal lumen is the following: (1) the dilution caused by osmotic attraction of water from the blood and (2) the movement of fluid from the lumen into the blood secondary to the transport of solutes.

If a hypotonic solution enters the intestine, the flux of water from lumen to blood is greater than from blood to lumen, leading to net absorption of fluid. This in turn is followed by the isotonic uptake of fluid.

The gut normally absorbs all electrolytes and water presented to it and, unlike the kidney, does not appear subject to hour-by-hour homeostatic regulation. Nevertheless, some external regulation occurs. The autonomic nervous system has effects on NaCl transport. Adrenergic (α-receptor) or anticholinergic stimuli tend to increase absorption, but cholinergic or antiadrenergic stimuli tend to decrease absorption. Other agents (e.g., serotonin, dopamine, the endogenous opiates, enkephalins, and endorphins) alter gut transport, usually in the secretory direction. However, the opiates morphine and codeine increase gut absorption.

The ileum has relatively little ability to respond to Na^+ depletion and/or mineralocorticoids. By contrast the large intestine is sensitive to both these assaults, which can increase Na^+ absorption and K^+ secretion. Mineralocorticoids can decrease the Na^+ concentration in fecal water from 30 to 2 mEq/L and increase the K^+ concentration from 75 to 150 mEq/L. The influence of aldosterone on sodium transport is exerted at two points. There is an increase in Na^+ permeability of the brush border membrane caused by the activation of new sodium channels. Also, aldosterone apparently increases the number of Na^+ pump molecules in the basolateral membrane.

Factors that cause the osmotic retention of water in the gut lumen or stimulate fluid secretion may lead to diarrhea. Saline laxatives such as Epsom salts (magnesium sulfate [$MgSO_4$]) increase fecal water because of the slow and incomplete absorption of polyvalent ions. Disease states such as disaccharidase deficiency or monosaccharide malabsorption cause **osmotic diarrhea.**

INTESTINAL SECRETION

Both the small and the large intestines secrete water and electrolytes. This process resides primarily in the crypt cells and is responsible for maintaining a liquid chyme.

The transcellular secretion of Cl^- accounts for most of the secretory activity, and the mechanism is illustrated in Figure 12-5. Cl^- enters the cell through a carrier located in the basolateral membrane. The carrier uses the Na^+ gradient established by the Na^+,K^+-ATPase to move Cl^- into the cell against its electrochemical gradient. Two Cl^- are moved into the cell along with one Na^+ and one K^+ via this $NaKCl_2$ cotransporter. The Na^+ entering the cell is extruded by the Na^+ pump, and K^+ diffuses back out of the cell through chloride

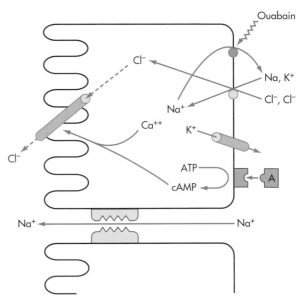

FIGURE 12-5 ■ Model for the secretion of Cl^- and Na^+ by the crypt cells of the small and large intestines.

channels in the apical membrane. Na^+ moves through paracellular pathways, driven by the lumen-negative potential difference created by the secretion of Cl^-. The resulting secretion of Na^+ and Cl^- establishes an osmotic gradient that draws water into the lumen.

The apical membranes of the crypt cells contain at least two different chloride channels. One is activated by increases in intracellular Ca^{++} and is stimulated by acetylcholine released by the enteric nervous system. The other type is stimulated by agents that increase cyclic adenosine monophosphate (cAMP) and is identical to the cystic fibrosis transmembrane conductance regulator (CFTR) that also is found in pancreatic and airway epithelial cells. Agents such as vasoactive intestinal peptide (VIP), secretin, and prostaglandin that stimulate this channel activate adenylate cyclase to increase cAMP, which in turn activates cAMP-dependent protein kinase A. Defects in this channel account for the intestinal, pulmonary, and pancreatic problems associated with cystic fibrosis.

Secretion that is stimulated by GI hormones and neurotransmitters after a meal is a physiologic aid to digestion, serving to maintain a liquid chyme during the process of absorption. However, excessive Cl^- secretion, with accompanying fluid secretion, can become pathologic in nature. The resulting **secretory diarrheas** are prevalent in many developing nations and constitute a leading cause of death. In some instances this disorder can be due to excessive blood levels of normal secretagogues such as VIP, which can be produced by certain tumors. In the great majority of cases, however, secretory diarrhea is caused by infection of the gut by pathogenic bacteria such as *Vibrio cholerae* and *Escherichia coli*. These bacteria produce enterotoxins that bind to receptors on the apical membranes of crypt cells. Receptor binding permanently activates the adenylate cyclase located on the basolateral membrane, and the cell is stimulated to secrete maximally for its lifetime. Huge volumes of water and electrolytes may be secreted, so that the absorptive capacity of the gut is greatly exceeded. Unless proper therapy is available, dehydration and death can result.

Ca++ ABSORPTION

Absorption of Ca++ by enterocytes is an important component in the regulation of whole-body Ca++ (Figure 12-6). The transepithelial movement of the cation occurs against an electrochemical potential. The process, although not entirely known, is localized in the proximal small intestine. Calcium transport occurs in four major steps. First, Ca++ absorption involves entry at the brush border membrane. Second, a mechanism must be present to regulate intracellular Ca++ levels to prevent altered cell function. Third, **vitamin D** affects at least one of these steps. Fourth, Ca++ exit occurs at the basolateral membrane. This section presents a scheme for calcium absorption compatible with these four points.

Transport of Ca++ is initiated by 1,25-dihydroxyvitamin D_3 [1,25-$(OH)_2$-D_3]. This active product is derived from vitamin D_3 (cholecalciferol) formed in the skin by the action of ultraviolet radiation on 7-dehydrocholesterol. Vitamin D_3 is transferred to the liver and converted to 25-OH-D_3. The kidney, through a step regulated by parathyroid hormone, converts 25-OH-D_3 to 1,25-$(OH)_2$-D_3. Enterocytes take up the 1,25-$(OH)_2$-D_3, where it reacts with a receptor molecule in either the nucleus or the cytosol (exact site unknown). The transcription of specific deoxyribonucleic acid (DNA) and protein synthesis are mandatory

FIGURE 12-6 ■ Calcium absorption by an enterocyte within a larger scheme of Ca++ homeostasis. Vitamin D_3, 1,25-$(OH)_2$-D_3, stimulates Ca++ transport by interacting with nuclear receptors to effect the synthesis of calcium-binding protein (CaBP). Ca++ enters the cell facilitated by brush border CaBP and exits via two mechanisms. It is speculated that CaBP in the cytosol stimulates Ca++-ATPase. Binding proteins in the Golgi, endoplasmic reticulum, and (possibly) mitochondria prevent a rise in intracellular Ca++ during the absorptive process. RNA, ribonucleic acid.

steps in the action of 1,25-$(OH)_2$-D_3 on Ca++ transport. The Ca++-binding activity of the synthesized protein correlates with Ca++ transport. Presumably at least one calcium-binding protein (CaBP) is inserted into the brush border and facilitates (gates) the entry of Ca++ down an electrochemical gradient.

Once inside the cell, CaBPs found in the Golgi apparatus and endoplasmic reticulum minimize the rise in intracellular free Ca++. It has been proposed, but not substantiated, that the mitochondria participate in this "buffering" action. This binding of Ca++ by the Golgi apparatus may possibly be a 1,25-$(OH)_2$-D_3–dependent process.

Exit of Ca++ at the basolateral membrane is against an electrochemical gradient and involves two mechanisms.

The more important mechanism is the Ca^{++}-ATPase, which may be 1,25-(OH)$_2$-D$_3$–dependent. The other is an Na$^+$-Ca^{++} exchanger, which functions when the Ca^{++}-ATPase is saturated.

Calcium absorption is regulated over the long term by plasma Ca^{++} levels. As intestinal absorption of Ca^{++} rises, plasma Ca^{++} increases; this change inhibits the secretion of parathyroid hormone. In turn, formation of 1,25-(OH)$_2$-D$_3$ in the kidney is inhibited (see Figure 12-6). A reduction in 1,25-(OH)$_2$-D$_3$ will eventually cause Ca^{++} absorption to wane, because the synthesis of new CaBP will cease. Although the mechanism of Ca^{++} absorption is not a closed issue, the model depicted in Figure 12-6 provides a currently popular working hypothesis.

IRON ABSORPTION

Absorption of iron is regulated by total body iron requirements and by the bioavailability of iron. Under physiologic conditions, dietary iron is acquired through transport processes in the proximal small intestine. Although the stomach, ileum, and colon have some capacity for iron absorption, this process is most prevalent in the duodenum and jejunum. Normally, because body iron is conserved, absorption of iron by the gut is low compared with the amount ingested.

Heme (derived from meat) is an important dietary source of iron. After it is absorbed intact by enterocytes, it loses iron from its porphyrin ring. Heme is absorbed, probably by endocytosis, and digested by lysosomal enzymes to release free iron. In all other chemical forms, iron is absorbed only to the extent to which it can be released from food in ionizable form. The insoluble complexes of iron with food become more soluble at a low pH. Gastric acid is important in solubilizing iron, and patients with deficient acid secretion absorb less iron. Organic acids such as ascorbic or citric reduce Fe^{+++} to Fe^{++}, which is absorbed more efficiently. Nonheme iron represents the largest fraction of dietary iron, and its absorption is dealt with in the following discussion.

The cellular mechanism of iron transport has not been completely described. However, a working hypothesis can be synthesized from what is known about the influx of iron across the brush border, its intracellular processing, and its efflux across the basolateral membrane of enterocytes into the circulation (Figure 12-7).

The enterocytes of the proximal small bowel release an iron-binding protein called *transferrin*, which binds two ions in the lumen. The transferrin-iron complex is recognized and bound by receptors on the brush border membranes of the duodenum and jejunum. The complex is absorbed, the receptor is recycled, and the transferrin-iron complex is transported to the basolateral membrane. The iron appears in blood bound to plasma transferrin, which is a β$_1$-globulin similar, but not identical, to intestinal transferrin. The movement of iron out of the enterocyte is poorly understood.

Some iron is transferred rapidly into the circulation, while some is combined intracellularly with a specific protein, apoferritin, to form a complex called **ferritin**. A small amount of iron combined with ferritin can be taken up slowly by the body after conversion to free iron. However, most ferritin-bound iron is lost when the epithelial cell exfoliates. Iron transferred to the blood is transported through the cytosol to the basolateral membrane by a protein that conveys it to the intercellular space. The "transport protein" (intestinal transferrin) is similar, but not identical, to transferrin. The latter is

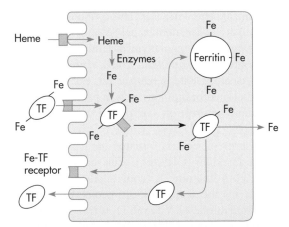

FIGURE 12-7 ■ Iron absorption. Iron absorbed as heme is freed within the cell by an enzymatic process and bound to transferrin (TF). Enterocytes secrete TF, which binds iron in the lumen. The complex is absorbed by a receptor-mediated process. Some iron is bound to ferritin and stored within the cell. Iron bound to TF enters the blood by an unknown process. The receptor is recycled, and TF can be resecreted.

a β_1-globulin that binds to iron as it exits the enterocyte and then transports it in plasma.

The body requirement for iron influences intestinal uptake. Absorption is thought to be regulated at a minimum of two sites. First, it depends on the binding of iron to brush border receptors, whose number is influenced by whole-body iron requirements. Second, it is regulated by the ratio of intracellular transport protein to storage protein (ferritin). The formation of ferritin is greatest when the body iron levels are high. Thus, iron transfer to the blood is low. The reverse holds during iron deficiency. For example, if iron depletion interferes with body functions such as hemoglobin synthesis, intestinal absorption of iron increases by the formation of more iron receptors on the brush border and by an increase in the intracellular iron transport protein relative to ferritin.

Systemic factors that control or regulate the rate of intestinal absorption of iron remain unknown. However, a feedback system has been proposed that entails both the transport and the storage of iron. Excess iron in the blood is carried to various body tissues, primarily the liver, where it is deposited as ferritin (storage iron), as it is in the intestinal mucosa. Ferritin-stored iron is in equilibrium with transferrin. During high storage conditions, transferrin in the plasma becomes saturated and can accept no more iron from parenchymal tissue stores or from mucosal cells. Thus iron absorption from the mucosa decreases. The existence of this feedback system and the factors that regulate the cellular mechanism of iron transport in the mucosa remain to be established.

SUMMARY

1. Approximately 9 L of water enters the GI tract per day. Of this amount, 2 L is ingested, and 7 L is secreted into the lumen. The small intestine absorbs about 8.5 L and the colon 0.4 L, leaving only 100 mL to be excreted in the stool.

2. The absorption of water occurs by diffusion down an osmotic gradient created by the absorption of Na^+, Cl^-, other electrolytes, and nutrients such as sugars and amino acids.

3. Four mechanisms account for the absorption of Na^+: passive diffusion, countertransport with H^+, cotransport with organic solutes (sugars and amino acids), and cotransport with Cl^-. The presence of these mechanisms varies along the length of the bowel.

4. Throughout the bowel, Cl^- is absorbed passively down its electrical gradient. In addition to being absorbed with Na^+, Cl^- is absorbed in the distal ileum and colon in exchange for HCO_3^-, which is secreted into the lumen and accounts for the alkalinity of stool water.

5. Crypt cells contain channels for Cl^- secretion in their apical membranes that respond to increases in cAMP. Various toxins, such as cholera toxin, and GI peptides, such as VIP, trigger secretion via this

mechanism, which depends on the Na^+,K^+-ATPase of the basolateral membrane.

6. The small intestine actively absorbs Ca^{++} by a process dependent on vitamin D, which stimulates the synthesis of a cytoplasmic CaBP and in turn facilitates the entry of Ca^{++} across the brush border membrane.

7. Iron is absorbed as both heme and inorganic iron. A transferrin is secreted into the lumen by the intestinal cells. Transferrin forms a complex with two iron ions; the complex is absorbed by receptor-mediated endocytosis. Iron is released into the interstitial fluid and appears in the blood bound to a different transferrin.

KEY WORDS AND CONCEPTS

- Transcellular pathways
- Paracellular pathways
- Tight junctions/zonulae occludens
- Electrogenic potential
- Osmotic diarrhea
- Secretory diarrhea
- Vitamin D
- Ferritin

REFERENCES

Binder HJ, Sandle GI: Electrolyte transport in the mammalian colon. In Johnson LR (ed): Physiology of the Gastrointestinal Tract, 3rd ed. New York, Raven Press, 1994.

Bronner F, Lipton J, Pansu D, et al: Molecular and transport effects of 1,25-dehydroxyvitamin-D_3 in rat duodenum. Fed Proc 41: 61-65, 1982.

Chang EB, Rao MC: Intestinal water and electrolyte transport: mechanisms of physiological and adaptive responses. In Johnson LR (ed): Physiology of the Gastrointestinal Tract, 3rd ed. New York, Raven Press, 1994.

Conrad ME: Iron absorption. In Johnson LR (ed): Physiology of the Gastrointestinal Tract, 2nd ed. New York, Raven Press, 1987.

Cooke HJ, Reddix RA: Neural regulation of intestinal electrolyte transport. In Johnson LR (ed): Physiology of the Gastrointestinal Tract, 3rd ed. New York, Raven Press, 1994.

Dharmsathaphorn K: Intestinal water and electrolyte transport. In Kelly WN (ed): Textbook of Internal Medicine. Philadelphia, JB Lippincott, 1989.

Montrose MH: Small intestine, absorption and secretion. In Johnson LR (ed): Encyclopedia of Gastroenterology vol 3. San Diego, Academic Press, 2004, pp 399-404.

Powell DW: Intestinal water and electrolyte transport. In Johnson LR (ed): Physiology of the Gastrointestinal Tract, 2nd ed. New York, Raven Press, 1987.

Schultz SG: Cellular models of epithelial ion transport. In Physiology of Membrane Disorders. New York, Plenum Press, 1986.

13

REGULATION OF FOOD INTAKE

LEONARD R. JOHNSON

The human species evolved during a time when the source of the next meal was highly uncertain. As a result, the gastrointestinal tract evolved to optimize the processing of ingested material when it became available. Receptive relaxation allows the stomach to accommodate large volumes with minimal increases in gastric pressure. Digestive enzymes are secreted in great excess. The secretion of pancreatic lipase, for example, must be reduced by at least 80% before steatorrhea occurs. There is significant overlap in the specificity of transport proteins or carries for the absorption of most amino acids. Indeed, even the absorptive surface of the small intestine can be reduced 60% to 70%, so long as sufficient ileum remains to reabsorb bile acids and to absorb vitamin B_{12}, before increased amounts of nutrients appear in the stool.

The result is that virtually all ingested carbohydrate, protein, and fat are broken down and absorbed. It is impossible to saturate the digestive and absorptive capacities of the gastrointestinal tract. This situation was advantageous when acquiring a meal was uncertain and also required an expenditure of calories in the form of exercise, but now that the nearest meal is available by opening the refrigerator door or, worse, pulling into the parking lot of the nearest convenience store or fast food restaurant, the result is an epidemic of obesity with its sequelae of diabetes, cardiovascular disease, and some forms of cancer.

At present, more than two thirds of Americans are overweight, and one fourth are classified as obese. As the current younger generation ages, the percentage of persons affected by obesity is expected to increase to 40% by 2010. At that time, or before, obesity will displace cigarette smoking as the number one health problem in the nation. In rare cases, obesity can be caused by a gene mutation, but in an overwhelming majority of instances, it is the result of a long-term imbalance between intake and expenditure of calories. These two quantities must remain equivalent to maintain body weight. Although a certain amount of weight control can be effected by increasing caloric expenditure in the form of exercise, the fact of the matter is that most of us overeat.

APPETITE CONTROL

In view of the recognized importance of normal body weight for maintaining health, an understanding of the mechanisms regulating food intake seems imperative. Current knowledge of the regulation of food intake is far from complete, however, and only in the past few years has sufficient evidence been accumulated for inclusion in a textbook of gastrointestinal physiology. In fact, knowledge about this aspect of the field lags far behind that on the topics covered in other chapters of this book. Another significant difference between this subject and those of the other chapters is that the regulation of food intake depends heavily on contributions from systems other than the digestive system—namely, the endocrine and nervous systems.

THE NERVOUS SYSTEM

Signals affecting food intake are integrated in the brain. These signals include emotions and learned behavior, as well as hormonal and neural input from the endocrine system and the gastrointestinal tract. Input provides information regarding total energy stores, as well as the presence of nutrients within the digestive tract. In addition, the vagus nerve relays input regarding gastric distention, secretory activity, and the release of various hormones from the stomach and duodenum.

Hypothalamus

Most of the integration of signals affecting food intake takes place in the **arcuate nucleus** of the hypothalamus. Two pathways exist: one inhibiting food intake and increasing metabolism, the other stimulating food intake and inhibiting metabolism (Figure 13-1). The **melanocortin** pathway is made up of appetite-inhibiting neurons containing pro-opiomelanocortin (POMC), which releases α-melanocyte-stimulating hormone (α-MSH). α-MSH binds melanocortin receptors (MC4), present on second-order neurons, to inhibit food intake and increase the rate of metabolism. The stimulation of feeding is provided by the **neuropeptide Y** (NPY) pathway. Hunger signals stimulate the release of NPY, which binds to Y_1 receptors to increase feeding behavior and the storage of calories. It would make little sense for both of these pathways to be operating at the same time, and the NPY system also releases agouti-related peptide (AgRP), which is an antagonist of the MC4 receptor. In addition, peptides that stimulate the melanocortin system inhibit the NPY system. Some cases of obesity in humans have been traced to mutations in the *POMC* and *MC4R* genes. Approximately 5% of cases of childhood obesity have been linked to *MC4R* mutations.

Enteric Nervous System and Vagus Nerve

The enteric nervous system plays a profound part in the regulation of gastrointestinal motility and secretion. Its receptors sense different chemicals present in foodstuffs, changes in muscle tension, and various peptides released from endocrine cells and nerves present in the gut. Approximately 75% of vagal fibers are afferent, and much of this information is relayed to vagal nuclei in the brain. In some cases this input causes an efferent signal also relayed by vagal nerves, resulting in a change in gut function—a so-called vagovagal reflex.

Most afferent vagal fibers pass through the nodose ganglion and terminate in the **nucleus tractus solitarius** (NTS) of the hindbrain. The hindbrain is able to regulate food intake in response to peripheral signals if input from higher centers is surgically eliminated. Several peptides that stimulate satiety and decrease feeding are known to activate receptors present on **vagal afferents**. In addition, the vagus relays signals initiated by distention of the stomach. Vagal signaling to the NTS is integrated with information received by the hypothalamus to produce the appropriate responses in feeding behavior and metabolism. Experiments in which vagal afferent activity was blocked either chemically or surgically have demonstrated the importance of this pathway in the overall regulation of food intake. In these studies, the inhibition of sham feeding by nutrient infusion was prevented; the amount of material in the stomach no longer influenced meal size; and the effects of satiety hormones were eliminated.

FIGURE 13-1 ■ Integration of signals regulating food intake and metabolism by the components of the arcuate nucleus of the hypothalamus.

THE ENDOCRINE SYSTEM

The endocrine system is concerned primarily with the long-term regulation of food intake and the maintenance of body weight. Normally, body weight is maintained within a relatively constant range over long periods of time despite changes in physical activity, metabolic demand, and caloric intake. For example, after an illness, humans increase food intake until lost weight is regained. Body weight then plateaus at or near the pre-illness level, and food intake returns to normal. The same phenomenon can be observed in animals that have been fasted or force-fed to cause weight loss or gain, respectively. In each case, when the animal is allowed to eat ad libitum, food intake either increases or decreases to bring body weight back to normal levels. Long-term appetite and body weight are now known to be regulated, at least in part, by hormones from the pancreas and adipose tissue. (Table 13-1 lists hormones believed to affect food intake in humans.)

Insulin

Insulin is produced by the β cells of the endocrine pancreas and regulates glucose uptake, the storage of absorbed nutrients, and caloric or energy balance. Insulin can be transported across the blood-brain barrier and binds to receptors present in areas of the hypothalamus that control food intake. In patients with type 1 diabetes mellitus, the absence of adequate insulin is associated with increased food intake. In rodents, administration of insulin to the brain reduces food intake, whereas similar administration of insulin antibodies increases feeding behavior and weight gain. Additional evidence indicates that insulin potentiates satiety factors released from gut endocrine cells.

Leptin

Until the 1990s, fat was believed to do little but store calories and act as an insulator. In 1994 the discovery of **leptin**, an appetite-suppressing hormone secreted by fat cells, started a new era of research involving fat and the control of food intake. Leptin receptors have been identified on neurons present in both pathways in the arcuate nucleus of the hypothalamus. The pathway producing the appetite-stimulating peptides NPY and AgRP is inhibited by leptin, and the pathway producing POMC, which inhibits food intake, is stimulated by leptin.

Leptin appears to be part of a negative feedback system for the regulation of food intake. Thus, as fat stores increase and more leptin is released, food intake is inhibited and energy expenditure is increased. The discovery of leptin created a great deal of optimism that it could be used to reduce food intake in obese persons, until it was shown that most obese persons

TABLE 13-1			
Hormones Most Likely to Affect Food Intake in Humans			
HORMONE	SOURCE	SITE OF ACTION	CLINICAL EFFECT
Insulin	Pancreatic β cells	Hypothalamus	↓ appetite ↑ metabolism
Leptin	Fat cells	Hypothalamus ↓ NPY, AgRP ↑ POMC	↓ appetite ↑ metabolism
CCK	I cells of duodenum	Vagal afferents	↓ appetite ↓ gastric emptying
PYY	L cells of ileum and colon	Hypothalamus ↓ NPY, AgRP ↑ POMC	↓ appetite ↑ metabolism
Ghrelin	Endocrine cells of the oxyntic gland area of the stomach	Hypothalamus ↑ NPY, AgRP Vagal afferents	↑ appetite ↓ metabolism

AgRP, agouti-related peptide; CCK, cholecystokinin; NPY, neuropeptide Y; POMC, pro-opiomelanocortin; PYY, peptide YY.

have high circulating levels of the hormone. Thus, although exogenous leptin reverses obesity in humans caused by its absence, leptin deficiency is not the usual reason for overeating and obesity. Leptin resistance in obese persons may be due to its failure to cross the blood-brain barrier and reach the hypothalamus. A recent study has indicated that triglycerides, which are elevated in obesity, inhibit the transport of leptin across the blood-brain barrier.

THE GASTROINTESTINAL SYSTEM

Endocrine cells lining the gastrointestinal tract are the source of several peptides known to regulate feeding behavior. Some act on vagal afferents, relaying information to the satiety center in the hindbrain. Others are transported through the blood-brain barrier and act directly on the hypothalamus. The information reaching these two centers is integrated into the overall satiety/hunger response.

Cholecystokinin

Cholecystokinin (CCK) was the first peptide shown to elicit satiety. In 1973 Smith, Young, and Gibbs showed that CCK injection caused rats to stop eating and begin grooming. This response occurred in animals with an open gastric fistula, excluding gastric distention as a stimulus. As discussed in Chapter 1, CCK is released from I cells in the duodenal mucosa in response to fat and protein digestion products. CCK presumably causes its inhibition of feeding by acting on vagal afferents, because its effects are reduced by vagotomy or by chemical destruction of the vagal afferents with capsaicin. The effect of CCK also is inhibited by lesions of the NTS. CCK_1 receptors are present on vagal afferents, strongly supporting the idea that the short-term regulation of prandial satiety is largely due to the release of CCK. One of the physiologic effects of CCK also is the inhibition of gastric emptying. This results in increased gastric distention and contributes to the satiety response. In humans, the infusion of CCK inhibits food intake and decreases feeding time, and the infusion of a CCK_1 receptor antagonist produces the opposite effects. The arcuate nucleus of the hypothalamus and the NTS of the hindbrain are connected by reciprocally projecting neurons. Thus, the long-term

effects of centrally acting leptin are potentiated by the short-term release of peripherally acting CCK.

Peptide YY

Peptide YY (PYY) is another candidate for a short-term satiety factor released from the gut. Like NPY, it is a member of the pancreatic polypeptide family and is produced as a 36–amino acid tyrosine containing peptide. PYY is released from enteroendocrine cells (L cells) of the ileum and colon by fat digestion products and may act to inhibit gastric emptying and secretion at the end of a meal. Circulating PYY reaches the hypothalamus via semipermeable capillaries of the median eminence to bind Y_2 receptors, inhibiting NPY neurons and releasing inhibition of POMC neurons. In humans, intravenous infusion of PYY in amounts yielding blood levels similar to those following a meal reduces food intake in both lean and obese persons. Of interest, obese persons have lower endogenous serum levels of PYY than those in control subjects of normal weight.

Ghrelin

Ghrelin is a 28–amino acid peptide secreted primarily by endocrine cells in the oxyntic gland area of the stomach. The observations that it binds to the growth hormone secretagogue receptor, stimulates the release of growth hormone, and increases the appetite have provoked considerable interest in it as a regulator of food intake. Plasma levels of ghrelin increase during fasting, peaking just before food intake begins or when the subject is expecting a meal, and fall within an hour of the start of feeding. In the hypothalamus, ghrelin stimulates neurons of the arcuate nucleus that express NPY. It also appears to exert some of its actions directly on gastric vagal afferents and on the dorsal vagal complex. Intravenous ghrelin increases food intake in persons of normal weight, but its role in obesity is uncertain. Ghrelin plasma levels are low in obese persons, increasing only after weight loss—suggesting that increased circulating levels of the hormone are not responsible for overeating. Additional evidence from animal experiments indicates that ghrelin inhibits the release of leptin and that leptin has a negative influence on ghrelin release. Because the negative effect of ghrelin on leptin release is stronger, it has been suggested that ghrelin initiates the feeding response.

Additional Peptides

Other peptides from the gastrointestinal tract have been shown to inhibit food intake and may have anorectic functions. Current research is in progress involving glucagon-like peptide 1 (GLP-1), oxyntomodulin (OXM), and pancreatic polypeptide (PP). In addition to inhibiting food intake, GLP-1 stimulates insulin release and inhibits gastric emptying. OXM, like GLP-1, is a product of the preproglucagon gene and has potent inhibitory effects on food intake in rodents. Its effects, however, are exerted on the arcuate nucleus, whereas those of GLP-1 are confined to the brainstem. PP reduces food intake in mice when administered peripherally, but central administration produces the opposite effect. In humans, PP inhibits the intake of food. Additional experiments are necessary to elucidate whether any of these peptides has a significant physiologic role in the regulation of caloric intake.

TREATMENT OF OBESITY

Figure 13-2 presents the most likely approximation of current knowledge regarding the treatment of obesity. The agents shown plus a number of others and/or their receptors are candidates for the development of drugs to treat obesity. Leptin is effective in treating the rare cases of leptin deficiency, but resistance to the drug in the more common forms of obesity limits its usefulness. Two drugs are currently licensed to cause loss of weight. One of these inhibits pancreatic lipase, resulting in maldigestion and malabsorption of fat. The resulting steatorrhea is an unpleasant side effect, and the effectiveness of the drug is limited. The other acts centrally to prevent the reuptake of serotonin and norepinephrine. It also may have adverse side effects, although it does reduce appetite.

With greater frequency, obese patients with related health problems are turning to surgery as a means to lose weight. Weight reduction, or bariatric, surgery has proved to be a successful and permanent solution for many persons. The first procedures put into general practice were designed to decrease the absorption of ingested food by bypassing most of the absorptive surface of the small bowel. In the most popular of these,

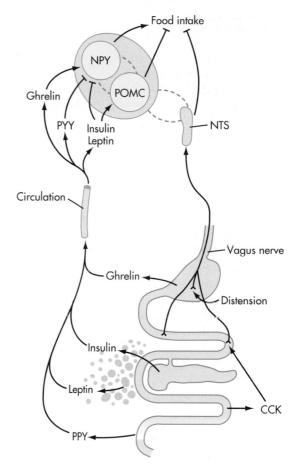

FIGURE 13-2 ■ Summary of mechanisms involved in the regulation of food intake. CCK, cholecystokinin; NPY, neuropeptide Y; NTS, nucleus tractus solitarius; PYY, peptide YY.

called jejunoileal bypass, the intestine was transected near the duodenal-jejunal border, the jejunal end was closed, and the duodenal end was anastomosed to the distal ileum. The problems caused by malabsorption, however, made this procedure undesirable.

Currently, gastric bypass is the most commonly performed procedure. A small gastric pouch is created to receive esophageal content. It in turn is connected directly to the small intestine, so that the storage function of the stomach is eliminated, reducing food intake.

SUMMARY

1. Obesity is rapidly becoming the number one health problem in the United States.
2. Our knowledge of the regulation of food intake is incomplete but has increased rapidly in the past 10 years or so.
3. Food intake is regulated by the nervous, endocrine, and gastrointestinal systems.
4. Satiety and hunger signals are integrated in centers in the arcuate nucleus of the hypothalamus and in the nucleus tractus solitarius of the hindbrain to regulate food intake and metabolism.
5. Long-term regulation is provided by the endocrine system in the form of insulin released from the pancreas and leptin released from fat cells. Both of these hormones inhibit the appetite, thereby limiting food intake.
6. Gastrointestinal peptides such as PYY, CCK and ghrelin are short-term regulators of food intake. PYY acts on the arcuate nucleus to suppress the appetite, whereas ghrelin acts on it to increase food intake. CCK and gastric distention activate vagal afferent fibers to the hindbrain to inhibit food intake and decrease the duration of a meal.

KEY WORDS AND CONCEPTS

- Arcuate nucleus
- Melanocortin
- Neuropeptide Y
- Nucleus tractus solitarius
- Vagal afferents
- Insulin
- Leptin
- Cholecystokinin
- Peptide YY
- Ghrelin

REFERENCES

Badman MK, Flier JS: The gut and energy balance: Visceral allies in the obesity wars. Science 307:1909-1914, 2005.

Blackman S: The enormity of obesity. Scientist May 24:20-24, 2004.

Konturek SJ, Konturek JW, Pawlik T, Brzozowski T: Brain-gut axis and its role in the control of food intake. J Physiol Pharmacol 55:137-154, 2004.

Rindi G, Torsello A, Locatelli V, Solcia E: Ghrelin expression and actions: A novel peptide from an old cell type of the diffuse endocrine system. Exp Biol Med 229:1007-1016, 2004.

Stephens P: The endocrinology of pediatric obesity. Endocr News October:24-27, 2004.

APPENDIX
Review Examination

MULTIPLE CHOICE

Select the best answer:

1. If a peptide belonging to the gastrin/cholecystokinin (CCK) family and having a sulfated tyrosyl residue in the seventh position from the C-terminus is desulfated, the most likely consequence for activity of the peptide will be
   a. a pattern of activity identical to that of gastrin.
   b. no change in pattern of activity.
   c. increased ability to stimulate gallbladder contraction.
   d. decreased ability to stimulate gastric acid secretion.
   e. a pattern of activity identical to that of CCK.

2. Gastrointestinal (GI) hormones
   a. stimulate their target cells from the luminal side of the gut.
   b. are for the most part inactivated as they pass through the liver.
   c. are released from discrete glands within the mucosa of the GI tract.
   d. pass through the liver and heart before reaching their targets.
   e. are bound to plasma proteins in the blood.

3. Cholecystokinin
   a. stimulates gastric emptying.
   b. is released by vagal stimulation.
   c. is released by protein and fat in the proximal small bowel.
   d. is released by distention when food enters the small bowel.
   e. is an important stimulator of gastric acid secretion.

4. Which of the following is *not* true about gastrinoma (Zollinger-Ellison syndrome)?
   a. Patients usually present with gastric ulcer.
   b. Patients develop diarrhea.
   c. Patients often have fat in their stools.
   d. Symptoms disappear after total gastrectomy.
   e. Following secretin injection, the levels of gastrin in the serum increase.

5. Stimulation of an intrinsic nerve in the intestine causes contraction of an intestinal muscle cell through the release of which neurotransmitter?
   a. Acetylcholine (ACh)
   b. Nitric oxide (NO)
   c. Norepinephrine
   d. Somatostatin
   e. Vasoactive intestinal peptide (VIP)

6. A nerve ending that releases NO onto a smooth muscle cell of the jejunum is injected with a dye that spreads throughout the nerve. The nerve cell body labeled by the dye most likely will be located in the
   a. brain.
   b. celiac ganglion.
   c. myenteric plexus.
   d. sacral region of the spinal cord.
   e. thoracic region of the spinal cord.

7. A muscle cell that has no striations and a ratio of thin to thick filaments of 15:1 most likely would be found in which region of the gastrointestinal tract?
   a. External anal sphincter
   b. Lower esophageal sphincter (LES)
   c. Pharynx
   d. Tongue
   e. Upper esophageal sphincter (UES)

8. In the presence of drug X, application of ACh to a bundle of gastric muscle cells causes membrane action potentials, an increase followed by a decrease in intracellular free calcium, but no contractile response. Drug X most likely is inhibiting which step in the contraction-relaxation process?
   a. Activation of myosin light chain kinase
   b. Binding of ACh with membrane receptors

143

c. Opening of membrane calcium channels

d. Opening of sarcoplasmic reticulum calcium channels

e. Spread of excitation among muscle cells

9. A lesion is made that results in loss of primary peristaltic contractions of the pharynx and esophagus, but secondary peristalsis of the lower esophagus occurs on distention of the esophageal body. The lesion most likely is in the
   a. cortical region of the brain.
   b. cricopharyngeal muscle.
   c. enteric nerves.
   d. nucleus ambiguus of the vagus.
   e. pharyngeal muscle.

10. A segment of esophagus is removed and placed in a tissue bath. The circular muscle in the segment contracts tonically and relaxes on stimulation of the nerves intrinsic to the segment. The segment is most likely from which region of the esophagus?
    a. Distal body of the esophagus
    b. LES
    c. Middle body of the esophagus
    d. Proximal body of the esophagus
    e. UES

11. A catheter that monitors pressure at its tip is inserted through the nose and passed an unknown distance. Between swallows it records a pressure that is subatmospheric and fluctuates during the respiratory cycle, decreasing during inspiration and increasing during expiration. In which region is the catheter tip most likely located?
    a. Esophageal body above the diaphragm
    b. Esophageal body below the diaphragm
    c. LES
    d. Orad region of the stomach
    e. UES

12. A patient experiences gastric "fullness" after eating only a small quantity of food. Manometry reveals normal peristalsis in both the upper and lower esophagus, but no receptive relaxation of the orad stomach. These findings are best explained by a defect in the
    a. nucleus ambiguus of the brainstem.
    b. dorsal motor nucleus of the brainstem.
    c. vagal nerves.

d. enteric nerves.

e. celiac ganglion.

13. Contractions of the orad stomach, proximal and distal antrum, pylorus, and proximal duodenum are monitored in a subject during the emptying of two meals that are identical except for their fat content. Compared with the low-fat meal, the meal high in fat would elicit
    a. a decrease in the force of pyloric contractions.
    b. an increase in the force of peristaltic antral contractions.
    c. an increase in the number of peristaltic antral contractions.
    d. an increase in the number of segmenting duodenal contractions.
    e. an increase in the number of tonic contractions of the orad stomach.

14. Slow waves are recorded from the orad stomach, proximal and distal antrum, and proximal duodenum in a fasted subject. Slow waves recorded during the burst phase of the migrating motor complex (MMC), compared with slow waves recorded during the relaxed phase, are characterized by
    a. a decrease in the apparent propagation velocity of antral slow waves.
    b. a decrease in the frequency of duodenal slow waves.
    c. an increase in the amplitude of antral slow waves.
    d. an increase in the frequency of antral slow waves.
    e. the occurrence of slow waves in the orad stomach.

15. Compared with the gastric motility response to a meal in an individual with intact vagus nerves, the response in an individual whose vagus nerves have been cut at a level just above the diaphragm would be characterized by
    a. decreased emptying rate of liquids.
    b. decreased emptying rate of solids.
    c. increased accommodation of the meal.
    d. increased mechanical reduction of food particle size.
    e. increased mixing of contents.

16. The rate of gastric emptying of a mixed meal of solid foods and liquids would be decreased by
    a. blocking activation of receptors in the duodenal mucosa.

b. enhanced tonic contraction of the orad stomach.

c. infusing an isotonic solution of sodium chloride into the duodenum.

d. infusing an isotonic solution of sodium chloride into the stomach.

e. infusing an isotonic solution of sodium oleate into the duodenum.

17. A patient experiences a rapid rate of transit of contents from the duodenum to the cecum. What characteristic would contractions recorded at various loci of the small intestine exhibit during this time?
    a. Frequency greater than that of the slow wave
    b. Low in force
    c. Mostly peristaltic
    d. Mostly segmenting
    e. Mostly tonic

18. Intravenous injection of a hormone initiates a phase of intense sequential contractions of the proximal duodenum that appears to migrate slowly toward the cecum. Which hormone was most likely injected?
    a. CCK
    b. Gastrin
    c. Motilin
    d. Secretin
    e. VIP

19. A region of the intestine contracts weakly on stimulation of its extrinsic nerves. Distention of the region elicits a peristaltic reflex, but with weak contractions. Slow wave activity is absent. Taken together, these findings suggest a disorder of the
    a. enteric nerves.
    b. parasympathetic nerves.
    c. release of motilin.
    d. smooth muscle cells.
    e. sympathetic nerves.

20. A normal subject's small intestinal contractions are recorded from three loci spaced 5 cm apart. Over a period of 2 hours, contractions occur at each site seemingly at random, with the interval between any two contractions being 5 seconds or a multiple of 5 seconds. Only rarely do contractions at the three loci seem to be in sequence. These data indicate that
    a. contractions are being recorded from the ileum.
    b. the subject is in a fasted state.

c. every slow wave is being accompanied by a contraction.

d. the contractions are causing rapid aboral transit of contents.

e. the contractions are mostly of the segmenting type.

21. Intraluminal pressure is monitored from a region of the colon that exhibits a relatively constant resting pressure of about 20 mm Hg. When an adjacent region of the colon is distended, resting pressure falls to near 0 and then increases slowly back toward 20 mm Hg even though the distention persists. The region being monitored is most likely the
    a. ascending colon.
    b. external anal sphincter.
    c. ileocecal sphincter.
    d. internal anal sphincter.
    e. transverse colon.

22. Segmental contractions of the colon
    a. increase in frequency in response to increased circulating levels of epinephrine.
    b. occur more often than do peristaltic contractions of the colon.
    c. occur at a higher frequency in the sigmoid colon than in the rectum.
    d. occur at a frequency that is higher than that for slow waves in the same region.
    e. are accompanied by the loss of haustral markings.

23. Relaxation of the ileocecal sphincter will occur during each of the following *except*
    a. eating a meal.
    b. distention of the ileum.
    c. distention of the colon.
    d. injection of gastrin.
    e. injection of cholecystokinin (CCK).

24. In a patient in whom resting tone of the internal anal sphincter is normal, distention of the rectum induces normal relaxation of the internal anal sphincter, no change in tone of the external anal sphincter, and no sensation of the urge to defecate. These findings are consistent with the finding of damage to the
    a. enteric nerves.
    b. internal anal sphincter.

c. vagus nerve.

d. spinal cord.

e. transverse colon.

25. The digestive action of saliva on starch is due to
   a. lactoferrin.
   b. lingual lipase.
   c. ptyalin.
   d. kallikrein.
   e. bradykinin.

26. At high rates of secretion, compared with low rates, saliva would have a lower concentration of
   a. Na^+.
   b. water.
   c. Cl^-.
   d. HCO_3^-.

27. All of the following are characteristic of saliva *except* that
   a. it has a high K^+ concentration.
   b. there is a large volume of secretion relative to the weight of the glands.
   c. both parasympathetic and sympathetic stimulation increase its flow.
   d. it is hypotonic.
   e. it is primarily regulated by hormones.

28. Salivary secretion is inhibited by
   a. smell.
   b. taste.
   c. nausea.
   d. pressure of food in the mouth.
   e. sleep.

29. Which of the following substances or combinations will produce the highest rate of acid secretion? (Each compound is given at its half maximal dose.)
   a. Histamine
   b. Gastrin
   c. Gastrin plus secretin
   d. ACh
   e. Histamine plus gastrin

30. Acid secretion during the cephalic response to a meal
   a. fails to occur when the antrum is acidified.
   b. is triggered by the entrance of food into the stomach.
   c. is prevented by vagotomy.
   d. is inhibited by insulin injection.

e. is stimulated only by ACh acting on the parietal cells.

31. Following the administration of histamine to a fasting individual, all of the following will occur within the parietal cells *except*
   a. a decreased amount of tubulovesicles.
   b. increased carbonic anhydrase activity.
   c. increased H^+, K^+-adenosine triphosphatase (ATPase) activity.
   d. an increased number of mitochondria.
   e. an increased area devoted to the intracellular canaliculus.

32. According to the two-component hypothesis for gastric acid secretion, the H^+ concentration in gastric secretion increases with the rate of secretion because
   a. the volume of the oxyntic component increases.
   b. the concentration of H^+ being secreted by the parietal cells increases.
   c. the volume of the nonoxyntic component decreases.
   d. the secretion of Na^+ is inhibited.
   e. the secretion becomes hypertonic.

33. Antral gastrin release is stimulated by all of the following *except*
   a. bombesin gastrin-releasing peptide (GRP).
   b. ACh.
   c. fat in the stomach.
   d. protein digestion products in the stomach.
   e. distention of the antrum.

34. The presence of acid (pH <3) in the duodenum
   a. inhibits gastrin release via somatostatin.
   b. increases pancreatic bicarbonate secretion.
   c. decreases bile production.
   d. increases gastric acid secretion.
   e. inhibits pancreatic enzyme secretion.

35. In someone with a total absence of gastric parietal cells, one would expect to find each of the following *except*
   a. decreased digestion of dietary protein.
   b. decreased absorption of vitamin B_{12}.
   c. little or no pepsin activity.
   d. increased growth of gut bacteria.
   e. lower than normal pancreatic bicarbonate secretion.

36. Administration of a drug that blocks the H^+,K^+-ATPase of the parietal cells of a secreting stomach
    a. will have no effect on the volume of secretion.
    b. will increase the concentration of H^+ in the secretion.
    c. will decrease the concentration of Na^+ in the secretion.
    d. will decrease the pH of the gastric venous blood.
    e. will decrease the potential difference across the stomach.

37. The interruption of vagal afferent fibers from the stomach would
    a. decrease the acid secretory response to sham feeding.
    b. decrease the release of gastrin by digested protein.
    c. decrease acid secretion in response to distention.
    d. decrease the release of somatostatin.
    e. increase acid secretion in response to histamine.

38. Between meals when the stomach is empty of food
    a. it contains a large volume of juice with pH approximately equal to 5.
    b. gastrin release is inhibited by a strongly acidic solution.
    c. it contains a small volume of gastric juice with a pH near neutral.
    d. bombesin acts on the parietal cells to inhibit secretion.
    e. it secretes large volumes of weakly acidic juice.

39. During the cephalic phase
    a. secretin stimulates pepsin secretion.
    b. CCK stimulates pancreatic enzyme secretion.
    c. ACh stimulates the G cell to release gastrin.
    d. bombesin stimulates parietal cell secretion.
    e. ACh stimulates pancreatic enzyme secretion.

40. In humans maximal rates of pancreatic bicarbonate secretion in response to a meal are due to
    a. the effects of small amounts of secretin being potentiated by ACh and CCK.
    b. large amounts of secretin released from the duodenal mucosa.
    c. VIP acting on the ductule cells.
    d. potentiation between CCK and ACh released from vagovagal reflexes.

    e. potentiation between small amounts of secretin and gastrin.

41. Vagal stimulation
    a. potentiates the effect of CCK on pancreatic acinar cells.
    b. directly stimulates pancreatic enzyme secretion.
    c. releases CCK from the duodenal mucosa.
    d. inhibits the effect of secretin on pancreatic ductule cells.
    e. releases secretin from duodenal mucosa.

42. Pancreatic enzyme secretion
    a. contains enzymes for the digestion of fat and protein but not carbohydrate.
    b. is primarily stimulated by secretin.
    c. is stimulated by pancreatic polypeptide.
    d. originates from the ductule cells.
    e. occurs primarily during the intestinal phase of the secretory response.

43. Pancreatic bicarbonate
    a. is secreted primarily from acinar cells.
    b. is secreted in quantities approximately equal to those of gastric acid.
    c. is stimulated primarily during the gastric phase of digestion.
    d. secretion causes an increase in the pH of pancreatic venous blood.
    e. ion concentrations in pancreatic juice decrease with increasing rates of volume secretion.

44. Pancreatic enzymes
    a. are synthesized in response to a secretory stimulus.
    b. are stored in Golgi vesicles.
    c. are secreted in response to carbohydrate in the duodenum.
    d. are secreted in response to sham-feeding.
    e. are involved in the breakdown of disaccharides.

45. A sample of bile taken from the gallbladder is compared with a sample of bile collected as it is being secreted from the liver. Compared with hepatic bile, the gallbladder bile will differ in that its
    a. bile salt concentration will be less.
    b. cholesterol/bile salt ratio will be greater.
    c. osmolality will be greater.
    d. phospholipid concentration will be less.
    e. potassium concentration will be greater.

46. Bile acid A has a greater solubility in intestinal fluid than does bile acid B. Compared with bile acid B, bile acid A is more likely to be
    a. a secondary bile acid.
    b. a trihydroxy rather than a dihydroxy bile acid.
    c. absorbed passively in the jejunum.
    d. unconjugated.
    e. undissociated.

47. When the distal ileum is removed, there will be an increase in bile acid
    a. levels in hepatic venous blood.
    b. levels in portal venous blood.
    c. secretion by hepatocytes.
    d. storage in the gallbladder.
    e. synthesis by hepatocytes.

48. As the bile secreted by the hepatocytes flows through the hepatic ducts on the way to the gall-bladder, there is an increase in bile
    a. bicarbonate concentration.
    b. bilirubin content.
    c. chloride concentration.
    d. H^+ concentration.
    e. osmolality.

49. The rate of absorption of free galactose in the small intestine, initially occurring at a submaximal rate, would be
    a. increased by adding an equal amount of glucose to the lumen.
    b. decreased by adding amino acids to the lumen.
    c. decreased by adding fructose to the lumen.
    d. increased by the addition of trehalose to the lumen.
    e. decreased by hypoxia in the enterocytes.

50. Which of the following enzymes is located in the brush border and plays a role in protein digestion?
    a. α-Dextrinase
    b. Carboxypeptidase A
    c. Pepsin
    d. Enterokinase
    e. Lactase

51. Colipase facilitates fat assimilation by
    a. digesting triglycerides.
    b. transporting fatty acids across cell membranes.
    c. preventing the inactivation of lipase by bile salts.
    d. converting prolipase to lipase.

e. binding fatty acids and monoglycerides after they have been absorbed by the enterocytes.

52. Most medium-chain fatty acids do not appear in chylomicrons because
    a. they are not absorbed by enterocytes.
    b. they are not transported by fatty acid–binding proteins.
    c. they do not bind to apoproteins.
    d. triglycerides containing them are not digested by pancreatic lipase.
    e. they are absorbed directly into the blood.

53. In the absence of enterokinase, one would also expect a decrease in the activity of
    a. pepsin.
    b. lipase.
    c. chymotrypsin.
    d. amylase.
    e. sucrase.

54. Amino acids
    a. are primarily absorbed in the distal gut.
    b. are, for the most part, absorbed by passive mechanisms.
    c. compete with glucose for Na^+ during their absorption.
    d. appear in the blood more rapidly when presented to the gut as small peptides rather than as free amino acids.
    e. are produced in the lumen primarily by the action of endopeptidases.

55. Each of the following acts as a good emulsifying agent *except*
    a. cholesterol.
    b. bile salts.
    c. fatty acids.
    d. lecithin.
    e. dietary protein.

56. Colipase
    a. digests the ester link in 2-monoglycerides.
    b. is a brush border enzyme.
    c. has no enzymatic activity.
    d. lowers the pH optimum of pancreatic lipase to match that of duodenal contents.
    e. displaces pancreatic lipase from the surface of emulsion droplets.

57. The fact that patients with a congenital absence of one of the amino acid carriers do not become deficient in that amino acid is due to the fact that
 a. the amino acid is absorbed by passive diffusion.
 b. the amino acid can make use of other carriers.
 c. the amino acid is absorbed by facilitated diffusion.
 d. peptides containing the amino acid are absorbed by different carriers.
 e. the amino acid is an essential amino acid.

58. Within the enterocytes
 a. triglycerides are resynthesized in the smooth endoplasmic reticulum.
 b. chylomicrons are synthesized in the smooth endoplasmic reticulum.
 c. fatty acid–binding protein transports long-chain fatty acids to the Golgi apparatus.
 d. triglycerides are synthesized from medium- and short-chain fatty acids.
 e. the major triglyceride resynthesis pathway makes use of dietary glycerol.

59. Of the 8 to 10 L of H_2O entering the digestive tract per day
 a. only 100 to 200 mL is excreted in the stool.
 b. most comes from the diet (includes liquids).
 c. most is absorbed in the large intestine.
 d. gastric secretions contribute twice the volume of those from the pancreas.
 e. most is absorbed against its own concentration gradient.

60. In the small intestine, Na^+ is absorbed by each of the following processes *except*
 a. diffusion.
 b. coupled to amino acid absorption.
 c. coupled to galactose absorption.
 d. coupled to the transport of H^+ in the opposite direction.
 e. coupled to the absorption of HCO_3^-.

61. In the distal portion of the ileum
 a. most fatty acids are absorbed.
 b. Cl^- is absorbed in exchange for HCO_3^-.
 c. Na^+ absorption occurs primarily coupled to glucose and amino acids.
 d. intrinsic factor is secreted.
 e. K^+ is absorbed in exchange for Na^+.

62. In the small intestine each of the following is true regarding Cl^- absorption *except that*
 a. it occurs down its electrical gradient.
 b. it occurs in exchange for Na^+.
 c. it occurs in exchange for HCO_3^-.
 d. it will result in the absorption of water.
 e. it occurs along the entire length of the small bowel.

63. Osmotic diarrhea may be the result of each of the following *except*
 a. cholera.
 b. lactase deficiency.
 c. inactivation of pancreatic lipase.
 d. Zollinger-Ellison syndrome (gastrinoma).
 e. loss of mucosal surface area in the small intestine.

64. Secretion of Cl^- by the small intestine
 a. occurs in exchange for HCO_3^-.
 b. takes place primarily in the villous cells.
 c. is inhibited by ouabain.
 d. produces an osmotic diarrhea.
 e. depends on an ATPase in the brush border membrane.

65. In the splanchnic circulation
 a. portal vein blood flow exceeds hepatic vein blood flow by about 50%.
 b. portal vein blood flow exceeds hepatic artery blood flow by about 50%.
 c. celiac artery blood flow exceeds hepatic vein blood flow by about 50%.
 d. celiac artery blood flow exceeds hepatic artery blood flow by about 50%.
 e. hepatic vein blood flow exceeds hepatic artery blood flow by about 50%.

66. The digestive system
 a. weighs more than the rest of the body.
 b. weighs half as much as the rest of the body.
 c. stores more blood that can be mobilized during exercise than any other part of the body.
 d. stores less blood that can be mobilized during exercise than do the voluntary muscles.
 e. contains half of the resting blood volume in the entire body.

67. Splanchnic conductance
 a. equals the blood pressure gradient ÷ splanchnic blood flow.

b. increases during vasodilation.

c. decreases during vasodilation.

d. increases during vasoconstriction.

e. decreases when splanchnic blood flow increases and the pressure gradient remains unchanged.

68. The major function of
    a. arterioles is to permit oxygen exchange from blood to parenchymal cells.
    b. arterioles is to permit glucose exchange from blood to parenchymal cells.
    c. venules is to provide resistance to the flow of blood.
    d. venules is to store blood that can be mobilized during exercise and other stresses.
    e. capillaries is to offer resistance to blood flow.

69. Vasodilator agents that bind to vascular smooth muscle surface receptors
    a. decrease the cytosolic calcium concentration.
    b. decrease the cytosolic cyclic adenosine monophosphate (cAMP) concentration.
    c. decrease the cytosolic cyclic guanosine monophosphate (cGMP) concentration.
    d. increase calcium flux into the cytosol from the extracellular space.
    e. increase calcium release from the sarcoplasmic reticulum.

70. A vasoconstrictor agent such as angiotensin II
    a. activates phospholipase C hydrolysis of plasma membrane lipids to form inositol triphosphate (IP_3) and diacylglycerol.
    b. prompts increased Ca^{++} entry into the cell from the extracellular space.
    c. causes release of bound calcium from the sarcoplasmic reticulum.
    d. elevates cytosolic Ca^{++} concentrations.
    e. probably causes all of the above.

71. Elevation of the cytosolic Ca^{++} concentration above 10^{-6} M
    a. activates phosphatase conversion of myosin phosphate into myosin.
    b. frees calmodulin for binding to actin.
    c. leads to vascular muscle cell contraction involving the interaction of actin and myosin.
    d. inactivates myosin kinase.
    e. causes all of the above.

72. All of the following naturally occurring substances are vasodilator agents *except*
    a. calcitonin gene–related peptide (CGRP).
    b. VIP.
    c. ACh.
    d. NO.
    e. Ca^{++}.

73. All of the following naturally occurring substances are vasoconstrictor agents *except*
    a. norepinephrine (α-adrenergic receptor stimulation).
    b. angiotensin II.
    c. bradykinin.
    d. vasopressin.
    e. leukotrienes.

74. Factors that contribute to gut mucosal cell death in nonocclusive intestinal ischemia include
    a. increased cardiac output and mesenteric vasodilation.
    b. parasympathetic stimulation and release of CGRP.
    c. digitalis and angiotensin II release.
    d. failure of oxygen countercurrent exchange to develop in the villi.
    e. stability of lysosomal membranes.

MATCHING

    a. Gastrin
    b. CCK
    c. Somatostatin
    d. Secretin
    e. VIP
    f. Histamine

75. Inhibits gastrin release when antrum is acidified

76. Inhibits parietal cell secretion of acid when antrum is acidified

77. Stimulates growth of gastric mucosa

78. Released by gastrin and acts as a paracrine to stimulate acid secretion

79. Stimulates gallbladder contraction in response to fat in the duodenum

80. Stimulates intestinal secretion and relaxes smooth muscle

A N S W E R S

1. **A**	17. **C**	33. **C**	49. **E**	65. **D**
2. **D**	18. **C**	34. **B**	50. **D**	66. **C**
3. **C**	19. **D**	35. **A**	51. **C**	67. **B**
4. **A**	20. **E**	36. **D**	52. **B**	68. **D**
5. **A**	21. **D**	37. **C**	53. **C**	69. **A**
6. **C**	22. **B**	38. **B**	54. **D**	70. **E**
7. **B**	23. **C**	39. **E**	55. **A**	71. **C**
8. **A**	24. **D**	40. **A**	56. **C**	72. **E**
9. **D**	25. **C**	41. **B**	57. **D**	73. **C**
10. **B**	26. **B**	42. **E**	58. **A**	74. **C**
11. **A**	27. **E**	43. **B**	59. **A**	75. **C**
12. **C**	28. **E**	44. **D**	60. **E**	76. **C**
13. **D**	29. **E**	45. **E**	61. **B**	77. **A**
14. **C**	30. **C**	46. **B**	62. **B**	78. **F**
15. **B**	31. **D**	47. **E**	63. **A**	79. **B**
16. **E**	32. **A**	48. **A**	64. **C**	80. **E**

INDEX

A

Abetalipoproteinemia, 123
Absorption, 108-125, 127-135
  anatomy-function associations in,
    107-109, 108f, 109f
  carbohydrate, 109-114, 110f-113f
  description and overview of, 108-109,
    109f, 127-128
  electrolyte, 127-135, 128f-130f, 132f-134f
  fluid, 127, 131-132, 131f
  lipid, 118-123, 119f-121f
  mucosal membrane role in, 108, 109f
  protein, 114-118, 114f, 114t, 115t,
    116f, 117f
  transport mechanisms following,
    108-109, 109f
  vitamin, 123-124, 123t
Acetylcholine
  acid secretion regulated by, 72-73, 74-77f
  gastrointestinal regulation and, 14
  pancreatic enzyme regulation by, 89-90,
    92f, 93f
  pepsinogen stimulation by, 78-79, 79f
ACh. *See* Acetylcholine.
Achalasia, esophagus role in, 28-29
Acid. *See also* Amino acids; Stomach, acid
  secretion by.
  reflux of, 29
Acinus
  enzyme production by, 88-89, 88f, 90f,
    92f, 93f
  pancreatic, 85, 88f, 90f, 92f, 93f
  salivary gland role of, 58-59, 58f, 62f
Actin, smooth muscle role of, 17f, 18, 18f
Adenosine triphosphate
  acid secretion role of, 68
  smooth muscle contraction role of,
    18, 18f
Amine precursor uptake decarboxylation
  cells, 5
Amino acids, 115-118, 115t, 116f, 117f
  carrier systems for, 115-116, 115t
  malabsorption of, 116-118, 117f
  transport mechanisms for, 115-116,
    115t, 116f, 117f
Amylase, 110, 110f, 111f
  carbohydrates digested by, 110,
    110f, 111f
  saliva containing, 57-58, 108f

Amylopectin, 110
Amylose, 109-110
Anal canal, 49-50
  defecation role of, 52, 52f
  innervation of, 14f, 50
  intraluminal pressure in, 52, 52f
  rectosphincteric reflex in, 52, 53
  sphincters of, 14f, 49-50
  striated muscle of, 14f, 49
Anemia, pernicious, 80-82, 81t
Antihistamine, acid secretion inhibited
  by, 73
Appetite control
  food intake regulated by, 137-138, 138f
  nervous system role in, 137-138, 138f
Assimilation, 107-125, 127-135
  anatomy-function associations in,
    107-109, 108f, 109f
  carbohydrates in, 109-114, 110f-113f
  electrolytes in, 127-135, 128f-130f,
    132f-134f
  fluids in, 127, 131-132, 131f
  lipids in, 118-123, 119f-121f
  proteins in, 114-118, 114f, 114t, 115t,
    116f, 117f
  vitamins in, 123-124, 123t
ATP (adenosine triphosphate)
  smooth muscle contraction role of,
    18, 18f
  stomach acid secretion role of, 68
Auerbach plexus, small intestine role of, 41
Autonomic nervous system, 13, 14f
  large intestine role of, 49
  neurocrine role in, 14-15, 16f
  pancreas innervation by, 85, 90f, 92f
  salivary gland regulated by, 59, 60f,
    63-64, 64f
  small intestine role of, 14f, 41

B

Bacterial overgrowth syndrome, 123
Basolateral membrane, amino acid
  crossing of, 115t
Beta carotene, 123t, 124
Bicarbonate
  intestine containing, 128, 128f, 130f
  pancreatic secretion of, 85-88, 86f, 87f,
    90f, 102
  salivary gland role of, 59-63, 61f, 62f

Bile, 97-106
  acids of, 97-102
    chemistry of, 97-98, 98f
    hydrophilic vs. hydrophobic, 97-98
  constituents of, 97-99, 98f
  daily loss rate of, 100
  electrolytes in, 99, 102-104, 102f
  expulsion of, 104-105
  gallbladder storage of, 102-104, 102f, 103f
  intestine containing, 99-104, 100f,
    102f, 103f
  phospholipids of, 98-99, 98f
  pigments of, 99, 101, 101f
  recirculation of, 99-102, 101f-103f, 104
  secretion of, 99-102, 100f-103f
  transport of, 99-104, 100f, 102f, 103f
Bile acid-dependent secretion, 102, 102f
Bile acid-independent secretion, 102, 102f
Bile duct, 102, 104
  obstruction of, 105
Bilirubin, 101, 101f
  conjugated vs. unconjugated, 101, 101f
  reticuloendothelial production of,
    101, 101f
Blood cells, 101, 101f
Blood group substances, saliva
  containing, 63
Bolus
  anal canal with, 52, 52f
  ingestion and transport of, 23-27,
    24f, 26f
  small intestine affected by, 42
Bombesin, 9, 9t
  acid secretion stimulated by, 74-76,
    74f, 75f
Bowel. *See* Intestine.
Bradykinin, salivary gland role of, 63
Brain, appetite control center of, 138, 138f
Brainstem, swallowing center in, 23, 25f
Brush border, absorption role of, 107, 109f

C

CaBP (calcium-binding protein), 133, 133f
Cajal interstitial cells, 19, 19f, 31-32, 41
Calcium
  absorption of, 133-134, 133f
  parathyroid hormone effect on,
    133-134, 133f
  saliva with, 57

Calcium *(Continued)*
  smooth muscle contraction role of,
    18, 18f
  transport mechanisms for, 133-134, 133f
  vitamin D affecting, 133
Calcium-binding protein, 133, 133f
Canaliculus, parietal cell with, 68, 69f, 70f
"Candidate" hormones, gastrointestinal,
    1, 8-9, 8t
Carbohydrates
  absorption and assimilation of, 109-114,
    110f-113f
  daily intake of, 109-110
  dietary forms of, 109-110
  digestion of, 110, 110f, 111f
  malabsorption of, 112-114, 113f
  transport mechanisms for, 110-111,
    112f, 113f
Carboxyl ester lipase, 118
Carboxypeptidase, protein digested by,
    114-115, 114f, 114t
Carcinoid syndrome, 122
Carrier systems. *See* Transport
    mechanisms.
CCK. *See* Cholecystokinin.
Cecum, 49-51, 51f
  contractions of, 50-51, 50f, 51f
  ileocecal junction of, 49-51, 50f, 51f
  intraluminal pressure in, 50-51, 50f
CEL (carboxyl ester lipase), 118
Celiac disease, malabsorption related to,
    112, 113f
Cell membrane. *See also* Transport
    mechanisms.
  absorption role of, 108-109, 109f
  amino acid crossing of, 115-116, 115t
  electric potential in. *See* Potentials.
Cell(s)
  acinar. *See* Acinus.
  blood, 101, 101f
  chief, 67, 79, 79f
  crypt, 132, 132f
  ductule, 85, 86f, 92f
  enterochromaffin-like, 7, 73, 73f
  epithelial
    gastric mucous layer from, 69
    water absorption role of, 131, 131f
  G, 68, 74-76, 74f, 75f, 77f
  gastrin-producing, 68, 74-76, 74f, 75f, 77f
  goblet, 107
  interstitial, of Cajal, 19, 19f, 31-32, 41
  liver, 99-101, 100f
  myoepithelial, 58f, 59
  oxyntic, 67-68, 68f
  parietal, 67-68, 68f-70f, 72, 73f
  peptic, 67-68, 68f, 69, 79, 79f
  pyloric gland, 67-68, 68f
  smooth muscle, 16-17, 17f
  stem, 68
Cephalic phase
  pancreatic secretions in, 89, 90f
  stomach acid secretion in, 74, 74f, 77f

CFTR (cystic fibrosis transmembrane
    conductance regulator), 87
Chief cells, 67
  pepsinogen stimulation in, 79, 79f
Chloride, 128f
  pancreatic secretion of, 85-88, 86f, 87f
  salivary gland role of, 59-63, 61f, 62f
  secretory mechanisms for, 132-133, 132f
  stomach secretion with, 70f, 71-72, 72f
  transport mechanisms for, 129-130,
    129f, 130f
Cholecystokinin, 2-12
  actions and interactions of, 6-8, 6t, 7t
  chemical structure of, 3-5, 3f
  discovery of, 2
  distribution and release of, 5-6, 5f, 5t
  food intake regulation by, 139t, 140, 141f
  pancreatic enzyme regulation by, 89-93,
    92f, 93f
  stomach emptying inhibited by, 78
Cholesterol, 121f
  absorption of, 122
  bile containing, 98f, 99
  chemical structure of, 98f, 99
Cholesterol esterase, pancreatic, 119
Cholic acid
  bile containing, 97-98, 98f
  chemical structure of, 97-98, 98f
Chylomicrons, 122
Chyme, stomach emptying and, 35
Chymotrypsin, 114-115, 114t
Chymotrypsinogen, 114-115, 114f, 114t
Cimetidine, stomach acid secretion
    inhibited by, 73
Circulation
  bile recirculation role of, 99-101, 100f,
    101f, 103f
  enterohepatic, 99-101, 100f, 103f
  salivary gland blood supply in, 59, 60f
Cobalamin, 123t, 124
Colon. *See also* Intestine, large.
  anal canal region of, 49, 52, 52f
  anatomy of, 14f, 49-51, 50f, 51f
  ascending, 49, 50-51, 50f, 51f
  barium in, 51f
  contractions of, 50-52, 50f, 51f
  descending, 49, 51-52, 51f
  electrolyte content in, 127-128, 128f, 130f
  innervation of, 14f, 49-50, 53
  intraluminal pressure in, 50-51, 50f
  peristalsis role of, 50-53, 50f-52f
  rectal, 49, 52, 52f
  sigmoid, 49, 51-52, 51f
  sphincters of, 49, 52, 52f
  transverse, 49, 50f
  water content in, 127-128, 128f
Constipation, irritable bowel causing,
    53, 54
Contraction. *See also* Migrating motor
    complex; Peristalsis; Sphincter(s).
  smooth muscle in, 17-20, 18f, 19f
Cricopharyngeal muscle, 24, 24f, 25f, 27

Crypt cells, chloride channels in, 132, 132f
Current. *See also* Potentials.
  pacemaker, 19, 19f, 32
Cystic fibrosis
  lipid role in, 122
  pancreatic deficiency and, 94
  transmembrane conductance regulator
    in, 87, 94
Cystinuria, malabsorption role in,
    117, 117f

D
Defecation, 52, 52f
Diarrhea
  dehydration due to, 133
  infection causing, 133
  irritable bowel causing, 54
  lipid role in, 122
  osmotic, 132, 133
  pancreatic cholera causing, 10-11
  secretory, 133
Diffusion
  absorption role of, 108-109, 109f
  passive, 108-109, 109f
Digestion, 107-125
  adaptation responses in, 109
  carbohydrate, 110, 110f, 111f
  description and overview of,
    107-108, 108f
  enzyme sources for, 107-108, 108f
  lipid, 118-119, 119f
  luminal/cavital form of, 107
  membrane/contact form of, 108
  protein, 114-115, 114f, 114t, 117f
Diverticulum, 54
Dorsal motor nucleus, esophagus and, 25f
Dry mouth, 57, 64
Ductule cells, pancreatic, 85, 86f, 92f
Duodenal ulcer
  acid output in, 81, 81t
  formation of, 82
  Helicobacter pylori in, 81-82, 81t
  stomach secretion role in, 80-82, 81t
  treatment of, 82
Duodenum
  electrolyte content in, 127-128, 128f
  emptying sequence in, 34, 35f, 37f
  intraluminal pressure in, 34, 35f,
    37f, 42f
  migrating motor complex in, 45f
  sphincter of Oddi in, 100f, 102-104,
    102f, 103f
  stomach emptying inhibited by,
    77-78, 78f
  ulcer of, 80-82, 81t
  water content in, 127-128, 128f

E
Eating. *See* Appetite control; Food.
Elastase, protein digested by, 114-115,
    114f, 114t
Electric potential. *See* Potentials.

Electrolytes
    absorption of, 127-135, 128f-130f,
        132f-134f
    bile containing, 99, 102f, 103-104
    intestine containing, 127-135, 128f-130f,
        132f-134f
    pancreatic secretion with, 85-88, 86f,
        87f, 90f
    saliva containing, 59-63, 61f, 62f
    stomach secretion containing,
        71-72, 72f
    transport mechanisms for, 70-71, 70f,
        109f, 128-131, 129f-134f
Emotion, small intestine affected by, 44
Emulsification, fat droplets in, 118
Endocrine system. See Hormone(s).
Endocrines, regulatory role of, 14-15, 16f
Endopeptidases, 114, 114f, 114t
Endoplasmic reticulum, pancreatic cell
    with, 88, 88f
Enkephalins, neurocrine status of, 9-10, 9t
Enteric nervous system, 13-14, 14f, 15f
    appetite control role of, 138
    myenteric plexus in, 14, 15f
    submucosal plexus in, 14
Enterochromaffin-like cells, 7, 73, 73f
    histamine found in, 73, 73f
Enterocytes, 107
Enterogastrone. See also Gastric
        inhibitory peptide.
    stomach acid inhibition due to,
        77-78, 78f
Enteroglucagon
    actions and interactions of, 8t
    chemical structure of, 4, 4f
Enterohepatic circulation, 99-101,
    100f, 103f
Enterokinase, protein digested by, 114-115,
    114f, 114t
Enterooxyntin, 72
Enzymes
    carbohydrates affected by, 110-114,
        110f-113f
    digestive, 107-108, 108f
    lipid affected by, 118-119, 119f
    pancreatic, 85, 88-89, 88f
    protein affected by, 114f, 114t
    saliva containing, 57-58, 63, 108f
    sites of production of, 107-108, 108f
Epinephrine, small intestine affected by, 44
Epithelial cells
    gastric mucous layer from, 69
    salivary gland role of, 58f, 59
    water absorption role of, 131, 131f
Esophagus, 23-29
    acid reflux affecting, 29
    clinical aspects of, 28-29
    innervation of, 25f, 26-28, 27f
    muscle layers of, 23-25, 25f, 27f
    peristalsis in, 23-28, 24f-26f
    pressure within, 23-25, 26f
    spasm of, 29

Esophagus (Continued)
    sphincter of, 23-24, 24f-26f
        lower, 24, 25f, 26f
        upper, 24, 25f, 26f
    swallowing role of, 23-29, 24f, 25f
Esterase
    cholesterol, 119
    nonspecific, 119
Evolution, food intake patterns in, 137
Exopeptidases, 114, 114f, 114t
Extrinsic nervous system, 13-14, 14f

F
FABPs (fatty acid binding proteins), 121
Facial nerve, 60f
Fat. See Lipid(s).
Fat droplets, 118
Fatty acid-binding protein, 121
Feces
    electrolyte content in, 127, 128f
    fat content in, 122
    pigments in, 99, 102
    water content in, 127, 128f
    weight of, 127
Feeding. See Appetite control; Food.
Ferritin, iron bound to, 134, 134f
Filaments, smooth muscle, 17f
Fluid
    absorption and assimilation of, 127,
        131-132, 131f
    bidirectional flux of, 127
    gallbladder transport of, 103-104
    pancreatic secretion of, 85-86
    unstirred layer of, 108, 109f
    water as, 121-132, 127, 128f, 131f
Fluoride, saliva with, 57
Food, 137-142
    appetite control and, 137-138, 138f
    bile secretion affected by, 99
    components of, 35, 36f
    hormone response due to, 5-6, 5f, 5t,
        139-140, 139t
    intake regulation for, 137-141, 139t, 141f
    pancreatic response to, 89, 93-94
    sham feeding of, 89
    stomach emptying and, 35, 36f
Fructose
    absorption of, 110-112, 111f, 112f, 113f
    daily intake of, 109-110
    malabsorption of, 112-114, 113f
    transport mechanisms for, 111-112,
        112f, 113f

G
G 34 (big gastrin), 4-5
G 17 (little gastrin), 3-5, 3f
G cell (gastrin-producing cell), 68, 74-76,
    74f, 75f, 77f
Galactose, intolerance of, 112
Gallbladder
    bile storage in, 99, 102-104, 102f, 103f
    volume of, 103

Gallstone, 105
    bacterial infection role in, 105
    imaging of, 105
    pigment substance in, 105
Ganglia
    myenteric esophageal, 25f
    prevertebral, 14f
    submandibular, 60f
Gastric acid. See Stomach, acid
        secretion by.
Gastric bypass, 141
Gastric emptying. See Stomach,
        emptying of.
Gastric inhibitory peptide, 2-12
    actions and interactions of, 6-8, 6t, 7t
    chemical structure of, 4, 4f
    discovery of, 2-3
    distribution and release of, 5-6, 5f, 5t
    stomach acid secretion inhibited by,
        77-78, 78f
Gastric juice. See Stomach, acid
        secretion by.
Gastric phase
    pancreatic secretions in, 89, 90f
    stomach acid secretions in, 74-76,
        75f, 77f
Gastric reflux, esophagus in, 29
Gastric ulcer
    acid output in, 81, 81t
    Helicobacter pylori in, 81-82, 81t
    stomach secretion role in, 80-82, 81t
    treatment of, 82
Gastrin, 2-12
    acid secretion stimulated by, 72, 73f
    actions and interactions of, 6-8, 6t, 7t
    big (G 34), 4-5
    chemical structure of, 3-5, 3f
    discovery of, 2
    distribution and release of, 5-6, 5f, 5t
    histamine and, 72-73, 73f
    hypersecretion of, 10
    little (G 17), 3-5, 3f
    parietal cell release of, 72, 73f
    production of, 74-76, 74f, 75f, 77f
    somatostatin cell release of, 76, 76f, 77f
Gastrin II, 3, 3f
Gastrinoma, 10-11
Gastrin-producing cell, 68, 74-76, 74f,
    75f, 77f
Gastrin-releasing peptide, 9, 9t
    acid secretion stimulated by, 74, 74f, 76,
        76f, 77f
Gastroduodenal junction, 31
    description of, 31, 34
    intraluminal pressure in, 34, 35f
    stomach emptying sequence in, 34,
        35f, 36f
Gastroenterostomy, 37-38
Gastroileal reflex, 53
Gastrointestinal tract. See also specific
        portions, organs, and functions.
    absorption in. See Absorption.

Gastrointestinal tract *(Continued)*
  biliary system in. *See* Bile.
  digestion in. *See* Digestion.
  electrolytes in. *See* Electrolytes.
  enzymes of. *See* Enzymes.
  fluids in, 127, 131-132, 131f
  general characteristics of, 1-2
  hormones affecting, 139-141, 139t, 141f
  intestinal segments in. *See* Intestine.
  mucosa of. *See* Mucosa.
  muscles of, 16-21, 17f-19f
  nerves affecting, 13-16, 14f-16f, 138, 138f
  neurohumoral integration of, 15, 16f
  peptides affecting, 1-12, 3f-5f, 6t-9t,
    139t, 140-141
  regulation of, 1-21, 138-141
G-cell. *See* Gastrin-producing cell.
Ghrelin, food intake regulated by, 139t, 140
GI. *See* Gastrointestinal tract.
GIP. *See* Gastric inhibitory peptide.
Glottis, swallowing role of, 23, 24f
Glucagon
  chemical structure of, 4, 4f
  islets of Langerhans production of, 85
Glucagon-like peptide 1, 9
  food intake inhibited by, 141
Glucose
  absorption of, 110-112, 111f, 112f
  daily intake of, 109-110
  intolerance of, 112
  malabsorption of, 112-114, 113f
  transport mechanisms for, 111-112,
    112f, 113f
Glycocalyx, absorption role of, 109f
Glycogen, 110
Goblet cells, 107
GRP (gastrin-releasing peptide), 9, 9t
  acid secretion stimulated by, 74, 74f, 76,
    76f, 77f
Gut. *See* Intestine.

H

Hartnup disease, 117-118
Haustra, 49, 50f
Helicobacter pylori
  stomach mucosa affected by, 81-82, 81t
  ulcer due to, 81-82, 81t
Heme, iron derived from, 134
Hemoglobin
  bilirubin from, 101, 101f
  splitting of, 101
Hepatocytes, recirculation role of,
  99-101, 100f
Hindbrain, appetite control center and, 138
Hirschsprung's disease, 53
Histamine
  acid secretion stimulated by, 72-73, 73f
  paracrine status of, 10
Hormone(s). *See also* Peptides.
  gastrointestinal, 1-12, 139-141
    actions and interactions of, 6-8, 6t, 7t
    "candidate," 1, 8-9, 8t

Hormone(s) *(Continued)*
  chemical structure of, 3-5, 3f, 4f
  clinical aspects of, 10-11, 137, 141, 141f
  discovery process for, 2-5
  distribution and release of, 5-8, 5f, 5t,
    139-141, 139t, 141f
  tract regulation by, 1-12, 3f-5f, 6t-9t,
    139-141, 139t, 141f
  integration of regulatory pathways by,
    14-15, 16f, 85
  large intestine affected by, 49, 53
  pancreatic, 85, 139, 139t, 141f
  small intestine affected by, 46, 139-141,
    139t, 141f
  testing related to, 11
Hunger, appetite control center and,
  138, 138f
Hydrochloric acid
  ion transport related to, 70-71, 70f
  parietal cell secretion of, 68
Hydrogen ion, 67
  stomach secretion with, 70f, 71-72,
    72f, 81f
Hypothalamus, appetite control center of,
  138, 138f

I

ICCs (interstitial cells of Cajal), 19, 19f
  pacemaker current of, 19, 19f
  small intestine role of, 41
  stomach with, 31-32
Ileocecal junction, 49-51, 50f, 51f
  gastroileal reflex in, 53
  intraluminal pressure in, 50-51, 50f
  motility role of, 53
  sphincteric mechanism of, 50, 50f, 51f
Ileum
  barium in, 51f
  electrolyte content in, 127-128, 128f
  ileocecal junction of, 49-51, 50f, 51f
  intraluminal pressure in, 50-51, 50f
  water content in, 127-128, 128f
Immunoglobulin A, salivary binding of, 57
Infection
  diarrhea caused by, 133
  malabsorption related to, 112, 113f
Insulin, 139, 139t
  food intake regulation and, 139,
    139t, 141f
  islets of Langerhans production of, 85
Intercalated duct, salivary gland role of,
  58f, 59
Interstitial cells of Cajal, 19, 19f
  small intestine role of, 41
  stomach with, 31-32
Intestinal phase, pancreatic secretions in,
  89-92, 90f, 92f
Intestine, 41-55. *See also*
  Gastrointestinal tract.
  bile transport in, 99-101, 100f,
    102f, 103f
  electrolytes in. *See* Electrolytes.

Intestine *(Continued)*
  large, 49-55. *See also* Colon.
    anatomy of, 14f, 49-51, 50f, 51f
    clinical aspects of, 53-54
    innervation of, 14f, 49, 53
    mass movement in, 51, 51f
    motility control in, 50-53
    muscle layers of, 14f, 49, 53
    peristalsis role of, 50-53, 50f-52f
    testing related to, 54
  neurons of, 14, 15f
  osmotic equilibration in, 127-128, 128f
  small, 41-47
    clinical aspects of, 46-47
    content mixing in, 42, 44, 44f
    contractions of, 41-46, 42f-46f
    emotions affecting, 44
    hormones affecting, 46, 139-141,
      139t, 141f
    innervation of, 14f, 15f, 41
    intraluminal pressure in, 41-42, 42f, 43f
    motility of, 42-46, 44f-46f
    muscle layers of, 41
    peristalsis in, 42, 44, 44f
    slow waves in, 43-46, 43f-46f
    testing related to, 46-47
    water content in, 127-128, 128f
Intestino-intestinal reflex, 44
Intolerance
  galactose causing, 112
  glucose causing, 112
  lactose causing, 111f, 112
Intraluminal pressure. *See* Pressure
  (intraluminal).
Intrinsic factor, 67, 68
  binding of, 124
  pernicious anemia role of, 79-80
Intrinsic nervous system, 13-14, 14f
Intrinsic primary afferent neurons, 15f
Ions
  luminal fluid containing, 127-128, 128f
  salivary gland, 59-63, 61f, 62f
  transport of
    hydrochloric acid secretion and,
      70-71, 70f
    mechanisms for, 109f, 128-131,
      129f-134f
IPANs (intrinsic primary afferent
  neurons), 15f
Iron
  absorption of, 134-135, 134f
  dietary source of, 134
  storage of, 135
  transport mechanisms for, 134-135, 134f
Irritable bowel syndrome, 53-54
Islets of Langerhans
  glucagon production by, 85
  insulin production by, 85

J

Jacobsen's nerve, 60f
Jejunum, migrating motor complex in, 45f

K

Kallikrein, salivary gland role of, 63
Kerckring's folds, 107

L

Lactase, deficiency of, 111f, 112
Lactoferrin, salivary, 57
Lactose, 110, 111f
  daily intake of, 109
  intolerance to, 111f, 112
Large intestine. *See* Colon; Intestine, large.
Larynx, swallowing role of, 23, 24f
Law of the intestines, 42, 44
Laxatives, 132
LDL (low-density lipoprotein), 122
Lecithin
  bile containing, 98-99, 98f
  chemical structure of, 98-99, 98f
Leptin, food intake and, 139-141, 139t, 141f
Lipase
  carboxyl ester form of, 118
  gastric, 118-119
  glycerol ester form of, 118, 119
  lingual, 58
  pancreatic, 119, 121f
  saliva containing, 58
Lipid(s)
  assimilation of, 118-123, 119f-121f
  digestion of, 118-119
  droplets of, 118
  malabsorption of, 122-123
  transport mechanisms for, 119-122,
    120f, 121f
Lipoproteins, 122
  apolipoprotein with, 122
  chylomicron form of, 122
  low-density, 122
  very-low-density, 122
Liver, recirculation role of, 99-101, 100f,
    102f, 103f
Lymphatic drainage, 131, 131f
Lysozyme, salivary, 57

M

Malabsorption
  amino acids in, 116-118, 117f
  carbohydrate products in, 112-114, 113f
  lipid products in, 122-123
  protein products in, 117
Maltose, daily intake of, 109-110
Meat, iron derived from, 134
Megacolon, 53
Melanocortin, 138, 138f
Melanocyte-stimulating hormone, 138, 138f
Membrane. *See also* Cell membrane;
    Transport mechanisms.
  basement, 109f
  basolateral, 115t
  potential. *See* Potentials.
Micelles, 97, 120f
  critical concentration for, 97, 120
  lipid transport role of, 120, 120f, 121f

Microvilli, absorption role of, 107,
    108, 109f
Migrating motor complex, 8
  motilin effect on, 8
  small intestine role of, 43, 44f, 45f, 46
  stomach emptying role of, 36, 37f
Migrating myoelectric complex, 8
  small intestine role of, 15f
MMC. *See* Migrating motor complex.
Monoglyceride acylation pathway, 121
Motilin, 2-12
  actions and interactions of, 6-8, 6t, 7t
  discovery of, 3
  distribution and release of, 5f, 5t
Motor complex. *See* Migrating
    motor complex.
Mouth
  salivary function in, 57-58
  swallowing and, 23, 24f
MSH (melanocyte-stimulating hormone),
    138, 138f
Mucosa
  gastric
    barrier function of, 67-69, 68f, 69f
    damage to, 71, 81-82, 81f
    Helicobacter pylori affecting,
      81-82, 81t
    ion transport in, 70-71, 70f
    membrane potential difference of, 71
    morphology of, 67-69, 68f-70f
    secretory function in, 67-69, 68f-70f
    ulcer and, 80-82, 81t
  gastrointestinal
    absorption role of, 107-109, 109f
    hormone release from, 1
Mucus
  gastric barrier function of, 67-69, 68f-70f
  properties of, 79
  saliva containing, 57
Muscle. *See also* Smooth muscle.
  cricopharyngeal, 24, 24f, 25f, 27
  esophageal layers of, 23-25, 24f,
    25f, 27f
  gastric layers of, 31-32
  gastrointestinal tract regulation by,
    16-21, 17f-19f
  small intestine, layers of, 41
  striated, 14f, 16
    anal canal, 14f, 49
    esophageal, 24, 25f, 27f
    pharyngeal, 24, 25f
Myenteric ganglia, esophagus and, 25f
Myenteric plexus
  enteric nervous system with, 14, 15f
  large intestine role of, 49, 53
  small intestine role of, 41
Myoelectric complex, migrating, 8, 15f
Myoepithelial cells, salivary gland role of,
    58f, 59
Myosin, smooth muscle role of, 17f, 18, 18f
Myosin light chain kinase, 18f
Myosin light chain phosphatase, 18f

N

Nasopharynx, 23, 24f
Nervous system, 13-15
  appetite controlled by, 137-138, 138f
  autonomic. *See* Autonomic nervous
    system.
  enteric, 13-14, 14f, 15f, 138
  extrinsic, 13-14, 14f
  food intake regulated by, 137-138, 138f
  gastrointestinal tract regulation by, 13-
    16, 14f-16f
  parasympathetic, 13-14, 14f
  sympathetic, 13-14, 14f
Neurocrines, 1, 9-10, 9t
  autonomic nervous system with,
    14-15, 16f
  integration of regulatory pathways by,
    14-15, 16f
Neurons
  intestinal pathways of, 14, 15f
  intrinsic primary afferent, 15f
Neuropeptide Y, 141f
Neurotensin, 9
Neurotransmitters
  neurocrines as, 14-15, 16f
  small intestine role of, 41
Nexus, smooth muscle role of, 17f
Nitric oxide, autonomic nervous system
    role of, 15
Norepinephrine, gastrointestinal
    regulation and, 15
Nucleus ambiguous, 23, 25f
Nucleus tractus solitarius, appetite and,
    138, 141f

O

Obesity, 137, 141, 141f
  clinical factors related to, 137
  treatment of, 141, 141f
Obstruction
  bile duct affected by, 105
  small intestine with, 46
Opiate receptors, gastrointestinal, 9-10
Oral cavity
  salivary function in, 57-58
  swallowing role of, 23, 24f
Oropharynx, 23, 24f
Osmotic diarrhea, 132, 133
Osmotic equilibration, 127-128, 128f,
    131-132
Oxyntic gland cells, 67-68, 68f
  morphology of, 67-68, 68f

P

PACAP (pituitary adenylate cyclase-
    activating peptide), 10
Pacemaker current
  cells of Cajal generation of, 19, 19f
  gastric emptying and, 32
Pancreas, 85-95
  anatomy of, 85
  clinical aspects of, 104

Pancreas (*Continued*)
  innervation of, 85, 90f, 92f
  secretions of, 85-94, 86f-88f, 90f-93f
    cephalic phase in, 89, 90f
    daily output volume of, 85-86
    electrolytes in, 85-88, 86f, 87f, 90f
    enzymic, 85, 88-89, 88f, 115
    fluid in, 85-86
    gastric phase in, 89, 90f
    intestinal phase in, 89-92, 90f, 92f
    potentiation of, 92-93, 93f
    regulation of, 89-92, 90f, 92f
Pancreatic polypeptide, "candidate
  hormone" as, 8, 8t, 85
Pancreatitis, alcohol role in, 115
Pancreozymin, 2
Paracrines, 10-11
  integration of regulatory pathways by,
    14-15, 16f
Parasympathetic nervous system, 13-14, 14f
Parathyroid hormone, calcium affected by,
  133-134, 133f
Parietal cells, 67-68, 68f
  gastrin release from, 72, 73f
  morphology of, 67-68, 68f-70f
Parkinson's disease, excessive salivation in, 64
Parotid glands, 58, 60f
PAT (proton-dependent amino acid
  transporter) protein, 116
PD (potential difference), 130
Pelvic nerves, large intestine role of, 49
Pepsin, 67, 68, 69
  physiology of, 78-79, 79f
  protein digested by, 114, 114f, 114t
Pepsinogen, 68, 69
  activation of, 78-79, 79f
  regulation of, 78-79, 79f
Peptic cells, 67-68, 68f, 69
  stimulation of, 79, 79f
Peptic ulcer
  acid output in, 81, 81t
  Helicobacter pylori in, 81-82, 81t
  stomach secretion role in, 80-82, 81t
Peptidases, protein digested by, 114, 114f,
  114t, 117f
Peptides. *See also* Hormone(s).
  acid secretion stimulated by, 74, 74f, 76,
    76f, 77f
  food intake regulation by, 139t,
    140-141, 141f
  gastric inhibitory, 2-12, 77-78
  gastrin-releasing, 9, 9t, 74, 74f, 76, 76f, 77f
  gastrointestinal regulation by, 1-12,
    3f-5f, 6t-9t, 139t, 140-141
  large intestine affected by, 50, 53
  small intestine role of, 41, 46
  vasoactive intestinal
    autonomic nervous system role of, 15
    chemical structure of, 4, 4f
    neurocrine status of, 9, 9t
    pancreatic cholera role of, 10-11
  YY form of, 8-9, 8t, 139t, 140

Peristalsis. *See also* Migrating motor
  complex.
  esophageal, 23-28, 24f-26f
  gastric emptying role of, 32
  large intestine role in, 50-53, 50f-52f
  "law of the intestines" role of, 42, 44
  opiate receptor role in, 9-10, 9t
  primary vs. secondary, 26
  small intestine in, 42, 44f
Pernicious anemia, stomach secretion role
  in, 80-82, 81t
Pharynx, 23, 24f, 25f
Phosphatidic acid pathway, 121-122
Phospholipase, 119
Phospholipids, 121f
  bile containing, 98-99, 98f
Pigments, bile containing, 99, 101, 101f
Pituitary adenylate cyclase-activating
  peptide, 10
Plexus
  myenteric, 14, 15f
  submucosal, 14
Portal circulation, bile recirculation role
  of, 99-101, 100f, 101f, 103f
Potassium
  intestine containing, 128f
  pancreatic secretion of, 85-88, 86f, 87f
  salivary gland role of, 59-63, 61f, 62f
  stomach secretion with, 70f, 71-72, 72f
  transport mechanisms for, 130, 130f, 131
Potentials
  difference in, 130
  electrogenic, 129-130
  gastric mucosa with, 71
  ion transport role of, 129-130
  membrane, 71, 86, 129-130
  myoelectric complex and, 8, 15f
  pacemaker current and, 19, 19f, 32
  pancreatic duct with, 86
  small intestine with, 44, 46f
  spike, 34, 44, 46f
  stomach contractions with, 34
Potentiation
  pancreatic basis for, 92-93, 93f
  stomach acid secretion stimulated by, 73
Pressure (intraluminal)
  anal canal with, 52, 52f
  cecum with, 50-51, 50f
  colon with, 50-51, 50f
  duodenum with, 34, 35f, 37f, 42f
  esophageal, 23-25, 26f
  gastroduodenal junction with, 34, 35f
  ileocecal junction with, 50-51, 50f
  ileum with, 50-51, 50f
  pylorus with, 34, 35f
  small intestine with, 41-42, 42f, 43f
  stomach emptying with, 34, 35f, 37f
Protein
  absorption of, 114-118, 114f, 114t, 115t,
    116f, 117f
  calcium-binding form of, 133, 133f
  digestion of, 114-115, 114f, 114t

Protein (*Continued*)
  fatty acid-binding form of, 121
  malabsorption related to, 117-118, 117f
  PAT protein as, 116
  R protein as, 124
  transport mechanisms for, 115-116,
    115t, 116f, 117f
Proton-dependent amino acid
  transporters, 116
Ptyalin, 57-58
Pudendal nerve, 50
Pyloric gland cells, 67-68, 68f
Pyloro-oxyntic reflex, 75
Pyloroplasty, 37-38
Pyloropyloric reflex, 75
Pylorus, 31
  description of, 31, 34
  intraluminal pressure in, 34, 35f
  stomach emptying sequence in, 34,
    35f, 36f
Pyridoxine, 123t, 124

R
R proteins, 124
Receptors, opiate, 9-10
Rectosphincteric reflex, 52, 53
Rectum, 49-50, 50f
  defecation role of, 52, 52f
  innervation of, 14f, 50
Red blood cells, bilirubin from, 101, 101f
Reflex
  gastroileal, 53
  intestino-intestinal, 44
  pyloro-oxyntic, 75
  pyloropyloric, 75
  rectosphincteric, 52, 53
  vasovagal, 75, 89, 92f
Regulation
  appetite control as, 137-138, 138f
  food intake, 137-138, 138f
  gastrointestinal tract in, 1-21
    hormones in, 1-12, 3f-5f, 6t-9t
    integration of pathways for, 14-15, 16f
    muscles in, 16-21, 17f-19f
    nerves in, 13-16, 14f-16f, 138
    neurohumoral integration of, 15, 16f
    peptides in, 1-12, 3f-5f, 6t-9t
  pancreatic secretion in, 89-92, 90f, 92f
  salivary gland, 59, 60f, 63-64, 64f
  stomach emptying, 35-37, 36f, 37f
Reticuloendothelial system, 101, 101f
Retinol, 123t, 124
Riboflavin, 123t, 124
Rough endoplasmic reticulum, pancreatic,
  88-89, 88f

S
Saliva, 57-65, 108f
  composition of, 57-64, 108f
    inorganic, 59-63, 61f, 62f
    organic, 61f, 63
  daily volume of, 58

Saliva (Continued)
    electrolyte content in, 59-63, 61f, 62f
    enzymes in, 57-58, 63, 108f
    functions of, 57-58
    regulation of, 63-64, 64f
Salivary glands, 57-65, 108f
    anatomy of, 58-59, 60f, 108f
    blood supply to, 59, 60f
    clinical aspects of, 57, 64
    daily events affecting, 64, 64f
    electrolyte transport by, 59-63, 61f, 62f
    enzyme synthesis by, 57-58, 63, 108f
    innervation of, 58-59, 60f, 63-64, 64f
    regulation of, 59, 60f, 63-64, 64f
Salivon, 58-59, 58f, 62f
Sarcoplasmic reticulum, 17f
Satiety
    appetite control center and, 138, 138f
    cholecystokinin role in, 140
Secretin, 2-12
    actions and interactions of, 6-8, 6t, 7t
    chemical structure of, 4, 4f
    discovery of, 2
    distribution and release of, 5-6, 5f, 5t
    pancreatic enzyme regulation by, 89,
        92t, 93, 93t
    stomach acid inhibition due to,
        77-78, 78f
Secretory diarrhea, 133
Segmentation, small intestine in, 42
Serotonin
    autonomic nervous system role of, 15
    small intestine affected by, 44
Sham feeding, pancreatic response to, 89
Shunt fascicles, 49-50
Slow waves
    large intestine with, 53
    small intestine with, 43-46, 43f-46f
    smooth muscle in, 19-20, 19f
    stomach emptying and, 32-34, 33f, 34f
Small intestine. See Intestine, small.
Smooth muscle, 16-20
    anatomy and morphology of, 16-17,
        17f, 19f
    cell structure of, 16-17, 17f
    contraction of, 17-20, 18f, 19f
        biochemistry of, 18-19, 18f
        tonic vs. phasic, 17
    esophageal, 24, 25f, 27f
    fasciae of, 17
    gastric layers of, 31-32
    slow waves of, 19-20, 19f
    unitary, 17, 17f
Sodium
    intestinal content of, 128f
    pancreatic secretion of, 85-88, 86f, 87f
    salivary gland role of, 59-63, 61f, 62f
    secretory mechanisms for, 132-133, 132f
    stomach secretion with, 70f, 71-72, 72f
    transport mechanisms for, 129-130,
        129f, 130f
Sodium pump, 129-130, 129f

Somatostatin
    autonomic nervous system role of, 15
    gastrin release inhibited by, 76, 76f, 77f
    inhibitory role of, 10
    paracrine status of, 10
Spasm, esophageal, 29
Sphincter(s)
    anal canal, 14f, 49-50
    esophageal, 23-24, 24f-26f
    of Oddi, 100f, 102-104, 102f, 103f
Spike potentials
    small intestine with, 44, 46f
    stomach contractions with, 34
Spinal cord, prevertebral ganglia and, 14f
Starch. See also Carbohydrates.
    daily intake of, 109-110
    saliva action on, 57-58
Starling forces, 127, 128
Steatorrhea
    lipid role in, 123
    pancreatic deficiency with, 94
Stem cells
    mucous cell differentiation of, 68
    parietal cell differentiation of, 68
Stomach
    acid secretion by
        anatomy related to, 67-69, 68f-70f
        cephalic phase of, 74, 74f, 77f
        daily output of, 68, 81t
        electrolytes in, 71-72, 72f
        gastric phase of, 74-76, 75f, 77f
        gastrinoma role in, 10-11
        inhibition of, 77-78, 78f
        intestinal phase of, 76-77, 77f
        ion transport related to, 70-71, 70f
        negative feedback mechanism for,
            77-78, 78f
        pathology related to, 80-82, 81f, 81t
        physiology of, 67-68, 70-82,
            72f-79f, 81f
        stimulants of, 72-77, 73f-78f
    anatomic regions of, 28, 28f
        antrum, body, fundus in, 28, 28f, 68f
        caudad vs. orad, 28, 28f
        secretory function in, 67-69, 68f-70f
    emptying of, 31-39, 36f
        caudad contractions in, 32-34, 32f-
            34f, 36f, 37f
        clinical aspects of, 37-38
        gastroduodenal junction in, 34, 35f
        inhibition of, 77-78, 78f
        intraluminal pressure in, 34, 35f, 37f
        orad contractions in, 32, 37f
        proximal duodenum in, 34-35, 35f, 37f
        pylorus in, 34, 35f, 36f
        regulation of, 35-37, 36f, 37f
        retropulsion mixing in, 32, 33f
        slow waves in, 32-34, 33f, 34f
        testing related to, 38
    innervation of, 31
    muscle layers of, 31-32
    receptive relaxation in, 28, 28f, 36f

Stomach (Continued)
    swallowing effect on, 26f, 28-29, 28f
    ulcer disease and, 80-82, 81f, 81t
Stones, gallstone in, 105
Stool. See Feces.
Striated duct, salivary gland role of, 58f, 59
Stuart-Briegleb representation, 98f
Sublingual glands, 58, 60f
Submandibular glands, 58, 60f
Submucosal plexus, enteric nervous
        system with, 14
Substance P, autonomic nervous system
        role of, 15
Sucrase, 110
Sucrose, 109-110
Sugar. See also Carbohydrates.
    dietary forms of, 109-110
Swallowing, 23-29, 24f-26f
    esophagus role in, 23-29, 24f-26f
    sequential factors in, 23-29, 24f-26f, 28f
    stomach response to, 26f, 28-29, 28f
Swallowing center, 23, 25f, 27
Sympathetic nervous system, 13-14, 14f

T
Taeniae coli, 49, 50f
Taste buds, saliva cleansing of, 57
Thiamine, 123t, 124
Tight junctions, 109f, 128
Tongue, swallowing role of, 23, 24f
Transferrin, iron bound to, 134, 134f
Transport mechanisms
    absorption role of, 108-109, 109f, 115t
    amino acids in, 115-116, 115t, 117f
    carbohydrate products in, 110-111,
        112f, 113f
    electrolytes in, 109f, 128-135,
        129f-134f
    lipid products in, 119-122, 120f, 121f
    protein products in, 115-116, 115t,
        116f, 117f
    tight junction role in, 109f, 128
Trigeminal nerve, parotid gland and, 60f
Triglycerides, lipid assimilation and,
        118-123, 119f-121f
Trypsin
    pancreatitis caused by, 115
    protein digested by, 114-115, 114f, 114t
Trypsinogen, 114-115, 114f, 114t
    premature activation of, 115
Tubulovesicles, parietal cell with, 68,
        69f, 70f

U
Ulcer disease
    acid output in, 81, 81t
    Helicobacter pylori in, 81-82, 81t
    stomach secretion role in, 80-82, 81t
    treatment of, 82
Unstirred layer of fluid, 108, 109f
Urobilinogen, production of,
        101-102, 101f

V

Vagotomy, stomach emptying delay
        due to, 37
Vagus nerve
    appetite control role of, 138
    food intake regulated by, 138
    large intestine role of, 14f, 49
    pancreas innervated by, 85, 90f, 92f
    small intestine role of, 41
    stomach acid secretion role of, 74-75,
        74f, 76f
Vasoactive intestinal peptide
    autonomic nervous system role of, 15
    chemical structure of, 4, 4f
    neurocrine status of, 9, 9t
Vasoactive intestinal protein, 10-11
Vasovagal reflex
    pancreatic enzyme regulation by,
        75, 89, 92f
    stomach acid secretion and, 75

VIP (vasoactive intestinal protein), 10-11
Vitamin A, 123t, 124
Vitamin B1, 123t, 124
Vitamin B2, 123t, 124
Vitamin B6, 123t, 124
Vitamin B12, 123t, 124
Vitamin C, 124
Vitamin D, 123t, 124
Vitamin E, 123t, 124
Vitamin K, 123t, 124
Vitamins, 123-124
    fat soluble, 123t, 124
    transport mechanisms of, 123-124
    water soluble, 123-124, 123t
VLDL (very-low-density lipoprotein), 122

W

Water
    daily intake of, 127, 128f
    fecal weight and, 127

Water *(Continued)*
    fluid absorption role of, 121-132, 127,
        128f, 131f
    gallbladder transport of,
        103-104
    secretion of, 131-132
Whipple's disease, lipid role in, 123

X

Xerostomia, 57, 64

Z

Zollinger-Ellison syndrome
    gastrinoma in, 10
    stomach secretion role in,
        80-82, 81t
Zonulae occludentes (tight junctions),
        109f, 128
Zymogen granule, pancreatic cell with,
        88-89, 88f